NINE *lives*

ISBN 978-0-912887-66-1
Library of Congress Control Number 2020938372

Edited by Mark Schreiber
Cover and Book Design by Lauren Grosskopf

Pleasure Boat Studio books are available
through your favorite bookstore and through the following:
Baker & Taylor, Ingram, Amazon, bn.com &
PLEASURE BOAT STUDIO: A NONPROFIT LITERARY PRESS
WWW.PLEASUREBOATSTUDIO.COM
Seattle, Washington

For my daughters, LISETTE *&* ANNICE

NINE *lives*

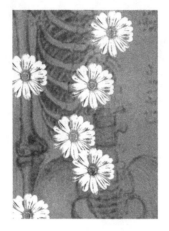

A NOVEL BY

DR. SIEGFRIED KRA

PLEASURE BOAT STUDIO: A LITERARY PRESS

CONTENTS

❖ *Prologue* ❖

THE WAITING ROOM was crowded with anxious patients waiting for me to arrive. One hour had passed, but they were expecting me to be late. As I paused outside the front door, I heard one man say: "He's always late, you know. He is in the hospital, but it's worth waiting for him."

"Don't you think?" said a woman in a loud voice. "Dr. Kra's a famous Yale professor with a very busy referral practice."

I entered the waiting room and waved to my patients with an apologetic smile. I then opened the door to my office secretary and said, "A little late sorry, Margo."

"You have lots of calls, doctor, from the hospital, and your father wants to speak to you."

I quickly looked over to the waiting room through the glass door that separated the waiting room from the offices and saw a number of new referrals. The walls of the waiting room were covered with paintings which I'd acquired from my visits to various museums around the world. The lithographs gave a bright, optimistic color to my practice. But there had been a time, in Danzig, when the paintings on the walls of my parents' estate were not reproductions.

I liked to think I had a charming smile and piercing brown eyes that twinkled when I was happy, and that women in particular liked my looks. I had a straight-looking body, muscular broad shoulders, a crop of gray hair, skin somewhat tanned, and a voice that was convincing and gentle if need be.

My private office was my pride. The floor covered with a large oriental rug, an expensive Tabriz, and an antique desk from 1860 accompanied by a swivel chair. A fragrant red rose sat in a Waterford glass on my desk. There were photographs on the wall of famous teachers and celebrity patients. There was also a picture of Danzig harbor with boats carrying coal and large signs reading, "BALTIC KOHLEN."

This had been my father's company before the Nazis invaded.

Today was the anniversary of my graduation from medical school. This was also the day my dear socialite mother died. She had a horrible disease called Scleroderma, that made her skin like parchment and her lungs like leather. Her heart was encased in a fibrous-like jacket. There was no treatment. Her beautiful delicate face soon looked like a character from a horror movie. She could not smile because her face was frozen in disease.

The Chief Resident in the Intensive Care unit had said, "We love your mother, but please tell her to be more cooperative. She will not allow us to examine her in the morning unless her hair is combed, lipstick on and wearing perfume."

I remembered when I visited her after my rounds at the hospital. She was in an oxygen tent, pulling the curtains away, not wishing to be in it.

"Don't do that! You need the oxygen to breathe!" I had yelled.

I left the Intensive Care unit after placing a kiss on her once beautiful face, now leather, and at three in the morning I got a call that she had suddenly died.

*

My last patient of the day was Hans Krause, an old family friend from Danzig. He had been referred from his family doctor because of palpitations and chest pain. After the usual questions, I took him to the stress lab for a cardiac stress test. Hans, who spoke English with a strong German accent, reminisced about Danzig.

"You were just a child, but I do remember you, believe it or not," he said as a he ran on the treadmill without even sweating.

"I will tell Father that you came to the office. I will see him this afternoon. There are not many people left from Danzig. Do you remember my mother, Lucy?"

"Of course, I remember her very well as that elegant woman. I heard she died. I did not escape to the U.S. like your family. I went to Argentina. We could not get a visa into United States. I'm here only for a short visit and then we'll return to Buenos Aires. Your father is a very smart man to have arranged for the escape. I was not Jewish, but still had to run because I did not sympathize with Hitler. Your father will tell you the whole story. I know you're a busy doctor now."

He finished his run on the treadmill. But now his face was red and then turned pale.

He whispered, "I don't feel right—something is going on."

He suddenly climbed off the treadmill and collapsed on the floor.

I pushed the Emergency bell.

I got on my knees and started CPR. The staff rushed in and swiftly placed leads from the defibrillator on his chest. I pushed the red button. An electric current surged through Hans' body and he almost became airborne.

He awoke and began speaking. "Oh, my chest is burning!"

His heart was in a regular rhythm and the blood pressure was normal. The CPR had been successful.

The ambulance arrived and took him to the hospital for observation.

"You guys did a great job," I complimented my well-trained nurses.

I had not anticipated that Hans would suffer an arrest, as his stress test was normal. But I had also recently reiterated to the residents at Yale New Haven Hospital, where I taught, not to be fooled by a normal test, as the arteries can still be blocked. I was used to cardiac emergencies in my office or the hospital, but I felt particularly uneasy from this experience, because with each passing year my connections to Danzig diminished.

I was busy with my last patient of the day when I got a call from the ER. I assumed it was about Hans, but it was a from a hospital in New York. My father had died from a heart attack.

"He was found lying on the street and died in the ambulance," I heard someone say.

"Can't be," I said. "He was healthy. I saw him last week. He looked great. We must get an autopsy!"

*

Jamaica Hospital was located in Queens, New York, adjacent to Highway 95. I took the train to Grand Central Station and the number five line subway to Queens. I had grown up in New York and often visited to see my father, go to shows on Broadway or opera at the Met, and visit museums.

I recalled my father once telling me he confronted a mugger by saying, "If the Russians could not kill me and Germans could not kill me, do you think you can, you hoodlum?" Then he pushed the gun out of the mugger's hand and ran him off.

*

I entered the Emergency Room with great trepidation. The hospital was located in a decrepit neighborhood with sidewalks covered with garbage and seedy-looking characters hanging around, leaning on broken down apartment buildings.

"I am Dr. Kra. My father, Henry Kra, was brought here this morning, and died. Is the doctor who saw him—is he still on duty?"

A minute later a tall dark man wearing a long white coat introduced himself as Dr. Gupta in a distinct Indian accent.

"I am sorry, doctor."

"Please tell me what happened."

"He arrived barely conscious, his heart was hardly beating. We struggled to put in a pacemaker. We tried CPR for twenty minutes then pronounce him dead."

"Can I see his ECGs?"

I sat in the doctors lounge to read them. I had read thousands of ECGs and now for the first time read my father's, wiping the tears from my eyes. I could not believe what I saw.

I suddenly ran out and spoke to Dr. Gupta in an angry voice, my face red and my eyes flashing with desperation.

"His ECG was normal! He did not have a heart attack. I demand an autopsy.

My father's body was still in the hospital morgue. So the officials decided to grant permission to perform an autopsy that very day after the Chief of Medicine and the Chief of Pathology agreed. I waited in the doctors lounge.

My father was a sturdy, strong man. At the age of 75 he was active and exercised daily. He had no history of heart disease. He was in the cavalry in Poland and fought the Russians in 1917.

*

The head nurse directed me to the patients office in the basement to pick up his belongings.

"My father, Henry Kra," I said in a quiet, sullen voice.

The clerk handed me his wallet, containing ten dollars, his apartment keys, and a pair of glasses. There were also his clothes: his shoes, suit, socks, shirt and tie. He must have gone to an appointment to be so dressed.

I walked towards the autopsy room, also in the basement. The pathologist greeted me with blood on his gloved hands.

"Well what did you find?" I asked impatiently, looking at my father's blood. "His heart was OK, but the belly was filled with blood. We will need a few days to find the cause," the pathologist informed me.

"What? So he did not die of a heart attack? And those idiots in the Emergency Room missed the diagnosis and wasted precious time trying to put in a pacemaker!"

*

I went to my father's building on Yellow Stone Boulevard in Queens and rode the elevator to the fifth floor. I felt like a burglar inserting the key. The familiar view and even the smells of the apartment made me want to yell out, "Hello, Father are you there?"

I walked through it with tears in my eyes. The small living room neatly furnished with a leather couch and four leather chairs in a semicircle resting on an oriental rug.

I walked into a second bedroom that served as his office. Old papers, photos of Danzig, and newspaper clippings were strewn on the desk. One picture of the *Queen Mary* was dated 1938, the year we sailed on her to the New World.

He had even kept the ticket stubs from the ship.

I sat down in his desk chair, remembering my parents and I standing together on the deck of the *Queen Mary* as we entered New York harbor.

Liberty

THE HMS *QUEEN MARY* slowed its engines as it sailed past the Statue of Liberty to dock in New York City. The passengers stood silently on the upper deck, some wearing fur collars and fur coats. These were the lucky ones who had escaped from the reign of terror of the Germans, who were on the verge of destroying an entire civilization. My parents and I had escaped from the Gestapo by boat from Danzig to Southampton in November, 1938.

The silence was broken by the jubilant playing of the Star Spangled Banner by the ship's orchestra. Some of the passengers stood wide-eyed, some cried, others applauded. Then, as the sun rose on the horizon, an apparition: suddenly I saw the magic city of tall buildings rising up from the sea like some great silvery monster.

I lifted myself on the railing below the pilot's deck to watch the burly men scurrying about the dock, tugging at the mass of ropes that secured the shifts.

Then came the loudspeaker announcing all refugees and passengers not holding American passports will depart from the AA Deck for customs inspections.

I found my parents in the long line that led to the gangplank.

"We were looking for you, get in line," my father said.

A large custom's inspector met us at the bottom of the stairs. "Welcome to the United States of America. Let's see your passports. Get your luggage please."

He pointed to a huge pile of suitcases on the pier, beside porters in blue uniforms waiting for their tips.

My father said, "No luggage. Only what we wear."

I smiled because I understood something that the porters were yelling. "Okay, okay!" I knew this word from the movies we saw aboard the *Queen Mary*, such as *The Adventures of Robin Hood*, with Errol Flynn.

I felt my short lederhosen to check if the money sewn in my pants was still there. When the custom's inspector glanced at me, I thought he could see right through my pants. But a minute later we were waved on and my mother pulled my hand as she hurried outside, where our wealthy American cousin waited to greet us.

*

Our rich American cousin checked us in to the Waldorf Hotel, where we stayed for two days before he found us an apartment on 89th Street and West End Avenue. But we barely heard from him after that.

My father looked for work but he spoke no English and America was suffering from a depression. Once a wealthy coal merchant and industrialist, he had no place in New York. He went to Blue Coal and many other companies, but they all refused him. We had no money except the coins sewn into my lederhosen. The Germans had taken everything away from us and we had to escape from the port of Danzig by fishing boat lest we end up in a concentration camp.

It had been impossible for us, or any Jews in German-occupied territory at that time, to get money out of our bank accounts, and we had millions. Fortunately my father had surreptitiously bought four tickets on the *Queen Mary* and arranged for our passports two years earlier. If only we had left then! But like so many others, my parents were convinced the Germans would come to their senses and Hitler would be but a footnote in history.

At the last moment, with the help of a boat captain who was a good friend, we escaped from Gdynia to Southampton, England and caught the *Queen Mary* to New York.

*

At the end of November it was quite cold. I was shivering, still dressed in short pants, as my mother insisted long pants were not for children.

She enrolled me in a public school on West End Avenue. The teacher, Mrs. Snyder, placed me in the first grade, a year behind, in a class for slow learners.

"I like *eis*," I said one day to the black boy who sat next to me in the lunch room.

The black boy pointed his finger at my eye and said, "You're eating an egg, not an eye."

I was using the German word for egg, called *ei*. My mother had packed a soft-boiled egg in my brown lunch bag. The egg was now spread over my face like an omelette. From my short pants I removed a small embroidered handkerchief and wiped my face. I left the apple and cookie in the brown bag and tossed it in the garbage pail.

I swiftly left the lunch room, my stomach growling, and mounted the two flights back to the classroom, humiliated, angry and hungry.

"You are back early," Mrs. Snyder said. "You can still stay in the cafeteria until the bell rings."

Just a few weeks before in Danzig I had sat in a class like this but facing a picture of Adolph Hitler and the Nazi flag. Now the American flag stood in the corner of the classroom. In Danzig there was no lunch period for me. The Jewish children were not allowed to go to school during the day, only in the afternoon.

*

During Geography class Mrs. Snyder took down a map of Europe. She said, "We have here a boy from Germany, from Danzig. He is a refugee."

She pointed to the place where I was born on the map, the Free State of Danzig, free no more.

The children all stared at me and laughed.

*

After school a tough-looking black boy came over to me, dropped his books, pushed me down and began to hit me in the face. I had learned to box at the Maccabee Club in Danzig and had no problem defending myself and retaliating with strong punches to the bully's face, until blood appeared from his nose.

"Hey man," the bully asked, wiping his bloody nose, "where did you learn to rumble like that? My name is Adolph," he continued, "Just call me Dolph. I like the way you rumble."

The bully-turned-friend gestured with his hand for me to follow him home. By now I had learned the way to go home on West End Avenue, a few blocks past Broadway. The other side of Broadway, the dangerous side, was Columbus Avenue, where Dolph was asking me to follow.

We arrived at a five-story apartment building. We entered a dark hallway that stank of urine and garbage.

He led me into his apartment, where a woman was standing, holding a baby. "This is my kid brother and my mother," Dolph said.

I had never seen a black woman, except in the movies at the art cinema in Danzig, where my Uncle Herman took me on Saturdays.

I tried not to stare at her.

Dolph said, "This is my first German friend. He don't speak English but he understands."

His mother gave me a pleasant smile. I bowed and clicked my heels. The light from the window showed a woman with a pleasant face who looked as though she'd just woken from a deep sleep. She seemed embarrassed to see me and quickly arranged her messy hair.

Dolph took me by the hand from the darkened room into the room adjacent.

"Here is where I sleep with my mother," he said.

There were two twin beds, each with a floral bed cover. The walls were bare with white, peeling paint.

Dolph then led me into another room, where he said his older brother sleeps. Then he took me up to the roof.

"Did you ever see a pussy?" he whispered.

He led me by hand to the edge of the roof and yelled to an open window across the street.

"Hey Shauna, show my new friend!"

A girl appeared in one of the windows below. She pulled down her panties and spread her legs apart.

I let go of Dolph's hand and swiftly ran downstairs and out of the building.

A Near Shipwreck

IN OCTOBER 1953 I received a letter admitting me to the Medical School in Toulouse, France.

Three days later, on a dreary morning, my parents drove me to the Brooklyn Naval Yard, where I boarded a tug boat to the *Mankato Victory* cargo ship, bound for Bremerhaven, Germany.

The tug boat swayed to and fro like the toy ships I had played with as a child in my bathtub in Danzig. The ocean was cold and the wind strong as the tug boat crawled to the ugly gray cargo ship.

A line was thrown by one of the tug boat crew and caught by one of the sailors on the cargo ship. A long ladder was then suspended from the top deck to the tug and I watched the crew hoist his trunk.

"You're next," the sailor called, as if I were just another piece of luggage.

I climbed in terror, hanging at times like a trapeze artist, as gusts of wind threatened to blow me into the sea. Once on top, two of the sailors were able to help me over.

"Pretty good, kid," one of them said.

The deck was crowded with military vehicles, jeeps and tanks. I was escorted through one of the steel entrances on the third deck to my cabin, located adjacent to the pilot room. My luggage was already in the room.

*

At 5:00 p.m. one of the sailors said dinner was being served in the galley. We were at sea already and it was dark and even windier than it had been in port. After several wrong tries, I finally found the galley, walking blindly up and down stairs.

Seated in the small area on wooden benches around a wooden table was the captain, the red-headed radio operator, the first mate, and the chief engineer.

A sumptuous meal of steaks and potatoes and ice cream was my first meal on the *Mankato Victory*. The captain had little to say. They ate quickly and returned to their duties. I went up to the deck and walked on the windy side and watched the rough sea and the bright stars. I missed my parents already, but felt like an adventurer on the high seas. Like Joseph Conrad.

*

Later I walked down to the deck where the crew hung out and found myself in a large narrow room where there was a strained table covered in cards and poker chips. The room was airless and filled with smoke, which seemed to bother only the medical student. They paid little heed to me, who thought it like a scene from *Heart of Darkness*, these rough able seamen arguing, shouting and laughing as if it were their last night on Earth.

I wandered back on deck as the Atlantic Ocean got rougher and the waves hit the *Mankato Victory* hard, making the ship roll side to side and the bow rise up, slamming down with a fierce force that made a loud booming sound.

I was allowed in the pilot's room and watched the angle of inclination showing deeper and deeper variations, as the first mate steered the ship. On deck were army vehicles bound for Iceland, our first destination. The weather got rougher, with water splashed over the deck. I slept fitfully that night, but was glad not to get seasick.

*

Two days later there was an even fiercer storm. I was in the radio room, talking with Sparkie, the Irish redhead, when he received an SOS that a cargo ship was in distress one hundred miles away, apparently split in half by the storm. But the *Mankato Victory* was itself struggling to stay above water. As the ship rolled violently the crew worked to secure ropes to aid in walking about the deck. The captain ordered me to return to my cabin.

But later I snuck up on the slippery deck, past the pilot's room where the captain and first mate were busy trying to keep the ship from breaking in two. The bow lurched up at a 45 degree angle. As I clutched onto the ropes, I watched in amazement as a tank broke loose and crashed into the truculent sea.

I saw the sailors rushing to secure the jeeps and offered to assist, but the captain screamed at me to get the hell off the deck.

*

Two nights later we arrived in Reykjavik, Iceland, lighter by the weight of a tank, but grateful to be alive, the ship seemingly no worse for wear.

I watched the jeeps being offloaded and then walked off the gangplank, past a statue of Leif Erickson, and into the nearest bar.

*

Four days later the *Mankato Victory* made port in Bremenhaven. I was awakened by a loud knock on my door. It was still dark and I thought this was a dream, or nightmare. Three tall men wearing black rubber raincoats with guns in holsters stood by the door speaking German.

"Border Police," one finally said in English.

I did not tell them that German was my native language. I had seen these faces before, in Danzig, except those men wore uniforms emblazoned with swastikas.

"I am an American," I declared, my voice weak and scared.

"Passport please."

I searched frantically through my suitcase, remembering my family's escape from Danzig Harbor, a lifetime before. I saw my childhood in flames, my uncles, aunts, cousins, friends marched into the gas chambers at Auschwitz.

"You were born in Danzig?" the officer asked, scrutinizing the passport.

"I am an American. A citizen of the United States," I said proudly, and fearfully.

The officer handed me back my passport. "Welcome to Germany."

War

I FOUND MY parents sitting on the couch facing the Emerson radio, listening to the Polish station. The announcer said Germany had bombed Danzig. My mother began to cry.

"We will now concentrate on becoming Americans," she said. "First learn English. And the boy must wear long pants."

*

Not that I needed long pants. The summer of 1939 was so hot you could fry an egg on the sidewalk. It was so hot that we sometimes spent our nights on the fire escape. We only had small fans. Even those with apartments facing the Hudson River suffered from the heat.

Some nights my parents and a few of their friends who had escaped from the Germans gathered on Riverside Drive, sitting on benches in a circle, singing and telling jokes in German, Polish and Yiddish until the early hours of the morning. I listened and fell asleep on a bench. These once-famous lawyers, scientists, artists, doctors, and businessmen like my father—the head of a large corporation—looked like vagabonds.

In the basement of our rooming house was a small store that pressed suits and shirts. The owner, a fat, ugly man, ran a thriving business. He had a son, Meurice, who delivered the suits, shirts and pants to the folks who lived on West End Avenue.

One day I was standing in front of the house when Meurice sized me up, looking at me curiously because I was wearing lederhosen on such a cold day.

"Why don't you wear long pants?" he asked.

I just smiled and Meurice became angry.

"Do you want me to punch you?" Meurice asked, growing angry. He raised his fist but at that moment his father emerged from the basement, wearing a stained polo shirt, a cigar dangling from his mouth, reeking sweat and alcohol.

"Meurice," he yelled. "Deliver these pants, damn you. He is a greenhorn. He does not speak English."

Meurice must have felt bad because he signaled me to follow him to the large apartment buildings on West End Avenue.

We entered a building through the servants elevator and rode to the twelfth floor. A black woman dressed in a white uniform answered the door. She took the clothes, paid the bill and gave Meurice a tip.

"See how easy it is?" he said, showing me the quarter in his palm.

*

The following afternoon after school I waited for Meurice in the basement. When Meurice arrived he was carrying a pair of long pants on a hanger.

"Here, this is for you. They're the same size as mine. Someone never came to pick them up. It's Christmas time and we can use help. My father will pay you 25 cents for delivery."

Of course I agreed. I was very happy to make this money, and so were my parents, despite the shame of the son of an industrialist doing menial labor. But we were lucky to eat one meal per day, usually noodles with sour cream, so this extra income significantly improved our diet.

Meurice and I became good friends after that.

*

During the day my parents listened to the small Emerson radio. In spite of Roosevelt being sort of isolationist to the terror rising in Europe, we greenhorns knew better. Germany was going to try to kill all the Jews. On the Polish station they heard that the Jews were dying from starvation, Typhus and random shootings by the Germans.

My father still had a gun that he brought with him on the *Queen Mary*, a Luger he kept in a drawer in his bedside table. It was loaded. He had used it in Danzig to defend himself when he was threatened by an S.S. officer. He shot him on a deserted road during a storm, and he only eluded arrest or assassination because of his connections in the civilian police.

*

On the corner of 99th and West End a group of well-dressed Jew-
ish-American boys hung out. They were several years older than me
and eyed me curiously, but without hostility, as I walked by.

They were pitching quarters against the sidewalk. The tallest of
the group asked me if he wanted to try. His name was Jack Tanne-
baum and he could tell I was a refugee. He gave me a quarter and told
me the object was to flip it as close to the wall as he could. I crouched
down and pinched it against the wall, hitting it flush. The boy I was
playing against landed his quarter farther out and all the boys but him
laughed loudly.

"Take it," Jack said to me. "You won."

This became another way for me to make money.

*

The following week I learned how to play marbles. The boys had beautiful looking marbles of different colors, which I'd never seen before.
Blue, purple, white, or clear. You could see through them like glass.

At that time you could buy a bag of marbles for ten cents, but they
weren't good quality and they couldn't be used for gambling. These,
however, were like gemstones and filled the bedroom closets of the
rich kids.

Jack showed me how to play. "Just bend down, flex your knees,
hold the marble gently between your finger and thumb and concentrate on the wall of the curb."

I mastered this game quickly and soon had my own large collection
of kaleidoscopic marbles, as well as rolls of quarters.

*

On December 7, 1941 we listened to the announcement on the radio
that the Japanese had bombed Pearl Harbor.

There was no more playing marbles or pitching quarters. The
Irish boys from Amsterdam Avenue started to attack me and my
Jewish friends after school. I had learned in Maccabee Club in
Danzig to stand against a wall during a fight so as not to be attacked
from behind. They came with stockings filled with rocks and sand,

swinging them as they found me, grabbing me by the neck, punching me everywhere.

I became good friends with a neighbor, Jerry Marshall, and we decided to defend ourselves, as there was no one to help us except Lionel, the black doorman, who would chase them off with a broom handle.

I got some lighter fluid and we poured it on paper airplanes, with wooden matches attached to the nose. When the planes crashed on the pavement the match would light. We climbed to the roof and waited for the hoodlums to come down the street. We then flung the planes and watched as they exploded into flames at their feet. The cowards took fright and did not bother us anymore.

*

As telephone calls were very expensive, Jerry and I took two paper ice cream cups, attached a very long string to each end and used them to talk to each other from our bedroom windows, or from the roof, where we would look out for the hoodlums.

One time Jerry's dog jumped off the roof, and after that my mother yelled at me for going up there, but she had never been much of a disciplinarian, so I ignored her.

*

Some of the rich Jewish boys turned in their marbles for playing cards and dice. They played poker and craps in the alleys behind the buildings, which were also used by men yelling up to have their knives sharpened, buying old clothes, and by opera singers serenading to get coins thrown down to them. One of the singers tore the string to our paper cups and that was the end of our phone.

*

With the war on there was a shortage of help, so Lionel, the doorman, showed me how to operate an elevator. For a dollar a day I ran the elevator after school and did my homework on the table in the wonderful old lobby.

In the next apartment building lived a family with two young children who needed a babysitter on the weekends. They asked me since I seemed responsible enough to run an elevator.

I gave most of my money to my mother.

*

Our landlord, whose name was Fineberg, would come each month to collect the rent. We were always two months late and had to borrow money from the Home Finance Company. The gas man came to shut the gas off so many times they knew us by name. My father was still struggling to earn money himself. He had no menial skills and he couldn't speak English. Our rich cousin must have appeased his own conscience by meeting us at the dock and helping us get settled, because he did nothing to help my father find a position in the New World.

So I became the family's breadwinner, finding ways to make money that presaged an entrepreneur or gambler more than a future cardiologist and writer.

One of my new enterprises cost me my babysitting job and another ended in a trip to the police station. A neighbor had a darkroom in the basement. He had taught me to process film before going into the army, and now I did this myself, at 20 cents a roll.

Meanwhile I was still babysitting. My friend Jack asked one day if he and his friends could use the apartment where I was babysitting to gamble. He offered me ten cents from each pot, which was a fortune in my eyes.

So on Saturday night after I tucked the kids in bed I gave the all clear to Jack and he brought up two folding bridge tables and a platoon of his Jewish gambler friends. I was told to stand lookout at the window while they played.

If that were all there was to it, just a few juvenile delinquents—future lawyers and bankers, and one cardiologist—playing poker on a Saturday night in New York City, no one would have called the police. Sure, I would have lost my babysitting job, and there would have been welts on our asses in the morning, but by the following week it would have all been forgotten, and I certainly wouldn't recall it all these years later.

What made this party singular was the fourteen-year-old Irish girl who appeared a little later at Jack's invitation. She didn't play poker, however, but was led into the parents' bedroom by Jack.

The parents came home early. I was in the bathroom and raced out with my fly still undone. We were completely surprised. The mother saw the two bridge tables with all these strange boys playing cards and screamed. But that was nothing compared to the father's yell when he opened his bedroom door and saw a girl spread-eagled on his bed.

I caught a glimpse of her naked body as she scampered for her clothes. The other boys gathered up the cards, money and tables and raced down the fire escape. I was left standing innocently in the center of the luxurious living room, which now looked like a tornado had swept through it.

"We thought you were a poor refugee," the father said, slapping me across the face. "Not a little gangster!"

*

My darkroom business also failed, but there was one last thing I was commissioned to do. One of the girls on West End Avenue was called Phoebe. Jerry, one of the gamblers, liked her. He was fifteen and she was thirteen. He got the idea to take a picture of his cock and send it to her with the note, "We want your ass."

He paid me a dollar to take the picture in the darkroom and develop it. That was the last I heard of the matter until two weeks later when the doorbell rang at two in the morning. I was sleeping, of course, but my mother had always been a nocturnal socialite and was awake reading the German-language papers.

I woke to the sound of her screams.

I peered out to see a uniformed policeman and a detective dressed in black, who reminded me of the Gestapo who had come to arrest us in Danzig. Had they traced us to New York?

"We are here to arrest a Siegfried Kra for sending erotic mail to Phoebe Nodelm," the detective informed my parents.

I came out, still in my pajamas and said I was Siegfried Kra.

My parents looked at me in shock. My mother knelt down and started asking a million questions, but my father told her in German not to say anything more.

She stayed behind while my father and I were escorted to the police station on Amsterdam Avenue. The detective led us into his office and told us to sit down. I was still in my pajamas and slippers, which fell off as I tried to touch the floor.

On the detective's desk was the picture of Jerry's cock, and the note.

"Son," he said, "do you know in America it is a federal offense to send pornography through the mail?"

I kept my eyes on the floor, at his fallen slippers. At that moment I was actually more afraid of my father than of the detective, who definitely was not the Gestapo. He has a pleasant voice and seemed to just be asking a question rather than accusing me of a capital offense. More than anything, I was ashamed to have brought disgrace upon my family in our new country.

"I didn't know," I stammered.

"Young man, what do you think Phoebe and her parents thought when they saw this?"

"I'm sorry. It wasn't my idea."

"We know," the detective said. "We have already talked to the other boy. But you took the picture, didn't you?"

"Yes."

"Are you allowed to take pictures like this and send them in the mail in your country?" he asked, more forcefully.

"*This* is my country," I told him, looking up.

The detective was nonplussed by such a patriotic answer, but the truth was I no longer thought of Danzig as my country, where simply being alive was punishable by death.

The detective put the photo and note in his ashtray, lit a match and dramatically set them on fire. Then he gave me a blank sheet of paper and a pen.

"Now you will write a note of apology to the girl and her parents. Does your father speak English?"

My father was still standing, erect like a soldier, with his hands clasped behind his back.

"A little," I answered.

The detective looked at my father while continuing to address me. "Tell him because you are so young there will be no charges pressed against you."

He waited for me to translate.

"But," he went on, "he and your mother need to keep a better eye on you. If you break the law again I will hold him accountable as well as you."

My father nodded to show he understood and clicked his heels.

Skeletons and Cadavers

THE TRAIN TO Paris arrived at Gare St. Lazarre. A former business associate of my father's whom I had never seen before was waiting for me on the platform.

I understood a little of his French as we drove in his car to Rue Charles V, where he lived on the top floor of an old building with his wife and son. He insisted I be on time to eat dinner at noon, a sumptuous four-course meal with wine.

I walked all over Paris with little money in my pocket and fell in love with the city. I was wishing and dreaming of having a girlfriend because Paris without love is a very lonely place. I passed famous cafes crowded with young Americans. I could only look with envy, lacking money even for a cup of coffee. No one bothered to talk to me as I walked along the Seine on the Left Bank, stopping at all the stalls packed with books and photos, hoping to find some of nude women.

At night I walked along side streets where the sewers ran open and the whores held court, trying to stop me. So many beautiful women. But I could only afford their smiles.

But I wasn't in France to fall in love. I was here to become a doctor. Medical school in the '50s was much cheaper in France than in the U.S., even factoring in transportation and lodging.

So after three days of falling in love with the sights, sounds, and especially the women of Paris, Pierre took me to the Gare Lyon station for the midnight Orient Express to Toulouse. Many years later I would take this train when it was revived as exclusively first class. But in the '50s there were three classes, and I travelled with the farmers and soldiers. There weren't any murders on this Orient Express, but I was almost asphyxiated by the putrid air and cheap cigarette smoke. On the train were French soldiers going to Algiers, as there was a war in North Africa under the command of French hero Charles De

Gaule, now President of France. It was a grim cold trip trying to sleep on the hard benches next to the soldiers who hadn't bathed in weeks.

*

Toulouse was a very old, famous city in the Midi France, on the Garrone River, not far from the Pyrenees. I found my way to a cheap hotel in the center where some of my compatriots were staying.

We were a group of American outcasts, unable to afford American medical schools, who made the Hotel Henri our new home. I had graduated from CCNY and been labeled a radical and a Communist, because I had participated in the riots in our school to oust an overtly anti-Semetic professor, one Dr. Knickerbocker. The Joe McCarthy years blackened many good people and produced hosts of casualties, but for me it was the beginning of an exciting new adventure.

Our small hotel was located one block away from the Place Capital, the center of the city, run with a warm hand by a gracious concierge and his wife, Madame and Monsieur Lelang. They lived in an apartment on the ground floor, immediately behind the circular desk of the lobby.

The rooms were small, but opened to an enclosed central court with a large circular skylight. There was a sink, a bed, a large armoire with a full-size mirror, and a small desk. Like all the other students, I had a miniature kerosene burner on which to brew coffee, fry eggs, and cook hamburgers in a cast iron pan. Although I had little money, given the inexpensive French bread, Camembert cheeses and wine, I made do with seventy dollars a month.

The concierge had no objections—at least none that he voiced— to my transformation of his room into an extension of the medical school. I decorated the walls and even the ceiling with paper blackboards, covered with formulas and detailed drawings of nerve connections for my anatomy class. This room became my sanctuary—at once my library, dining room, sleeping quarters and a place to dream of someday becoming a doctor.

Each morning a small elderly lady came to make the beds and sweep the best she could, especially the multi-colored chalk dust that covered the room and pervaded the air, intermingled with the odors of fried food, wine, and tobacco smoke from the night before. There was one large stained brown bathtub for each floor, for which we had to make reservations two days in advance. Weekends were the most desired reservations and, of course, the hardest to get. Madame Lelang ran a fair game and could not be bribed by the richer students to get first crack at this marvelous luxury. She provided soap and large woolly bath towels for the sumptuous and exhilarating experience. My room was moderately heated but the bathtub room was like a sauna.

Most of the students were considerably better off than I, and they frequently took their meals at one of the numerous nearby restaurants where the food was inexpensive but delicious. It was a luxury I could not afford. My fellow compatriots staying at the hotel included two rather introverted women on Fulbright scholarships who had come to learn French culture; one medical student from St. Croix, whose name was Ralph; a man from Brooklyn, Rosenberg by name, and Lionel Williams, from New York.

Rosenberg spoke French fluently because this was his second year in Toulouse, preparing to retake the tests he had flunked the first time. When he opened his room shutters, I could see a line of dried kosher salamis hanging in his open armoire. Each week they arrived, much like the newspapers, promptly and without fail. Bringing salamis to France is much like bringing a sandwich to the Cote Basque restaurant in New York. But this hardly concerned Rosenberg. His room looked and smelled like a New York delicatessen when he fried his treasured salamis on his kerosene stove. Salami and eggs—fit for the gods on Olympus, he thought.

You could always tell Ralph, the St. Croix native, was near by his cough. It echoed throughout the night because he kept his shutters opened. A mild and gentle man, he spoke French fluently. He too was in his second year in Toulouse, having also flunked his exams. He always had a cigarette in his hand, holding it like Peter Lorre, at the center, between his thumb and index finger, raising his hand, palm up, to meet his lips whenever he took a puff.

The oldest of the group was Lionel, a black man from New York City who had a wife and two children living in Harlem. All his life he had wanted to become a doctor. Now with grown children, his wife had to remain in New York, working hard and sending him money to enable him to pursue his dream. It was his first month here and he knew little, if any, French. He had been away from school for more than twenty years. Heavyset and tall, with a shiny face and a warm smile, Lionel was affable. He and I quickly became friends. We shared common bonds: New York, poverty, little knowledge of French, and our first time in Toulouse. Lionel was a decent and generous man with a vision of a golden tomorrow.

Whenever he cooked meatballs and spaghetti he shared his meal with me. In the mornings we left together for the bus at the Place Esquirole, which would take us the ancient Toulouse medical school, with its long marble staircases and the anatomy laboratory which dated back centuries.

*

In November, after our first two months at the school, the dissections of human bodies were performed. Twelve rectangular slabs were covered with gray corpses, men and women. At first Lionel and I gasped with astonishment to see so many dead, and I could tell he was disturbed at the thought that they were about to be mutilated. Lionel was a deeply religious man. Each night before going to bed he read the Bible. Now, as he stood petrified, I saw him offer a silent prayer. We were assigned to the same corpse—an Algerian who had died of gunshot wounds. There was a hole in the center of his head, another in the chest.

In all, four students were assigned to each corpse. Lionel and I were to start on the leg. We could not understand the instructions the professor raced through in French. A young assistant who spoke a little English gave us some basic directions about how to proceed with this ghastly business. The dissection kits were old and rusty. At CCNY we had better tools for our frog and cat dissections. I held the scalpel in my hand, pointing at the skin. And then, for a second, I recalled the words of Macbeth: "Is this a dagger which I see before me/ The handle toward my hand? Come, let me clutch thee/ I have thee not, and yet I see thee still?"

The incision was made; the skin of the thigh was tough and resilient, as hard as leather. Fluid oozed out of the incision. The strong smell of formaldehyde made my eyes smart and tear. It is a smell I will never forget. These were old bodies, long frozen in the morgue. Now life came crawling out of the legs—hundreds of maggots swimming in the juices of decay. I felt faint, but the pungent odor somehow kept me from swooning.

"Clean the skin area and identify the arteries and nerves and carefully dissect them clean. Cut the main artery or nerve and you fail the course before it begins."

Those were the discomforting words of Professor Rouviere, a tall, threatening-looking man with black hair pasted down on his head. The other students at our table knew no English. One was Algerian, the other French. I marveled how adroitly they performed their task. Surely they were destined to be surgeons. The signs were there. How cool they seemed, while Lionel and I perspired.

All of us wore heavy rubber aprons. The other two standing next to us were so confident that they seemed almost indifferent to what they where doing. How could anyone be so indifferent to human flesh? Wasn't this corpse once alive? What had the man done, what had he been like? But now there was no name, just a number, 36660, and a gender designation, male. Cold but efficient.

I watched the despair in Lionel's eyes. He was the same age as the corpse, the remains of a man who was now nothing more than a harbor and restaurant for maggots and an instrument of learning. I wondered—not for the first time—if this was the right profession for me. Carefully, we moved the fat to one side and, finding the long gray nerve, began to clean it. Pull too hard, allow the slimy scalpel to slip and that slender thread would be sliced through.

*

When we left in the darkness of the night our bodies reeked with that smell of death, especially our hands. Once back in my room I quickly stripped off the offensive clothing, only to remember that there would be no washing machine, no bath to soak in. These clothes would remain my uniform. I'd have to live with the stench.

Sitting at my desk, the French anatomy text spread before me, I began the tedious task of translating into English. Then came the memorization. Thousands of pages to memorize for just one course, and then all those others to follow—and all in French! Small wonder most flunk the exams the first time. How did anyone pass?

Becoming increasingly despondent, surrounded by the smells which almost made me retch, I heard a gentle knock on a door. So many sounds came from that busy courtyard that I wasn't sure if the knock was intended for me. This time of the night it could only be Lionel bringing me a cup of tea, as he sometimes did. Then we would sit and talk about New York and his family, and his eyes would become moist. He was so terribly lonely that first month. The knock came again, more insistent, and I knew it was not Lionel.

Standing there was an apparition, a vision. My first thought was that the fumes of the formaldehyde must have gone to my head. She was the most beautiful woman I had ever seen. She was sleek and bright-eyed, vivacious and animated. She spoke first—in a voice I found adorable—as she saw the astonished look on my face. She must have detected the stench of the formaldehyde, I thought, but she didn't make a comment about it.

"I saw your light on," she said in French. "Do you smoke?" she asked in English, her accent totally delightful.

"Yes. Please come in."

The only chair in the room was covered with clothing. I stuffed the clothes into the drawers of the large armoire that took up a good part of the room and, rummaging around in there, found a pack of matches and handed them to her.

"You are an artist," she giggled, looking up at the ceiling covered with the anatomical drawings. I wanted to be surrounded by the names and the images so they would become as much a part of me as my arms and legs. The first thing I saw each morning was the arterial supply of the stomach, as it was drawn on the ceiling.

"No, I am a medical student!"

"Yes, I heard you were the new one in the hotel!"

Her perfume mingled with and then overcame the disgusting smell of the formaldehyde, or at least so it seemed to me.

"My name is Monique," she said, tilting her beautiful head slightly to the side. Her hair was brown and short, almost like a young boy's in prep school. She touched the side of her head and I saw that her fingernails were covered with a deep red polish.

"You are still studying," she said, "and it is so late. I will leave you to your work."

"No, no. I have had enough for tonight," I blurted. "Please." I closed the door behind her and she came over to my desk and peered at the anatomy text.

"It is all in French!" she said. "Do you read French, *un peu*, a little? I can help you, if you wish, in the evenings when you are back from your classes!"

This was surely a dream.

Her body was small, slender, a perfect match for her delicate head and arms. Unself-conscious, she sat on the unmade bed, smiling and fully comfortable. After a moment she rose, walked to the desk where I was sitting and leaned over me to peer at the book I still held. I touched the hair on my head and remembered these hands were covered with the stench of the dead.

"That is the *cuisse,* how you say?"

"Thigh."

"*Voila,* thigh. It is not pretty without the skin." She laughed seductively, and I became weak.

"I will come tomorrow again, and I will help you translate."

"You don't have to go."

"Oh *oui,* it is late and I must get my beauty sleep." She kissed me on the cheek and left the room.

For the rest of the night the room was filled with her perfume and I was filled with thoughts of her.

In Europe, the students were an elite group, almost always forgiven for their wild ways. If they got drunk the Toulousian would say, "Oh, *c'est un etudiant.*" They are students, what do you expect?

You could always tell a student in Europe in those glorious days of the fifties. Most were unshaven or bearded, wearing old worn clothing. There was an air of freedom about them. No one was required to go to classes; all the learning was up to the student. There were no guides, no rules, only the final exams, the brutal task which always lay ahead, never for an instant out of mind. A one-time shot at the golden ring of success at the end of the year. Most repeated the year. Sometimes they stayed for several years to pass that first year.

Once the first was passed, the next seemed easy.

American students were even more special because of our reputation, often accurate, of being rich. I was an exception to the rule, and no one would quite believe I had barely enough money to eat more than one meal a day. It was almost impossible to have any social life without cash. I was prepared to lead a life of loneliness and celibacy and to concentrate all my energies on preparing for and passing the exams.

The second home for the students was the cafe, a welcome reprieve from our small, dingy, usually cold and poorly-lit rooms. I went as often as I could to the cafe and nursed a cup of coffee for hours sometimes, undisturbed by any obsequious waiter. Here I heard French being spoken, and watched, with great envy, love at work. Smoke-filled cafes with students busily speaking, surrounded by young women, laughing, not paying much attention to an obvious-looking American. Then, when it looked hopeless to meet anyone, I walked the narrow streets back to my dreary hotel, through the foggy night. I was hopelessly in love with love. I carried a sweet melancholy in my soul.

All around me there was love. Even Rosenberg, the salami king, managed to have a girlfriend visit him. This hotel had such thin walls, especially the one in which I was interned, facing the court. All the sounds of the night entered them. Ralph coughed all night, and Rosenberg's carnal grunts pervaded the court like a bad porno movie.

Too excited to sleep, I worked late and finished memorizing the arteries and nerve supply to the leg.

Breakfast consisted, as almost always, of a cup of Nescafe, some French bread and butter, and a slice of Camembert. At five in the morning, most of the students were up and about, having already started their studies and continuing until it was time to catch the bus at eight.

Lionel was at my door at five-thirty, a walking corpse who was grinning affably.

"You had a guest at 1:00 a.m.," he said.

"Well, yes, a dream floated into my room," I told him.

For the rest of the day my thoughts were of Monique. At the lecture hall we sat on marble steps as the ambidextrous professor lectured on and drew the anatomy of the leg, using different colored chalks, one in each hand, to sketch in the arteries and the nerves. He used not a scrap of notes.

"Gentlemen, that is how you must know each inch of the body."

The lecture hall was half empty, which was hardly unusual since attendance was not required at any of the lectures, but only for work in the laboratories and the hospital.

Lionel was struggling to catch some of the words the professor spoke. The Toulousian speaks a special French, a wonderfully musical version. They also roll their R's, making it almost sound a bit like Italian.

With little sleep and being distracted by my fantasy of Monique, I heard little of the lecture, but once in the anatomy laboratory and at our post by the leg of the corpse, there was no time to daydream. Stress ruled. Lionel struggled fiercely with his dissection. I could see the frustration line his face.

Later we sat in the cafe sipping coffee. We were so exhausted that studying was simply not possible. The cafe on the Place de Capital was crowded with students smoking Gauloise cigarettes. I had a few packs of milder Phillip Morris cigarettes in my room that I dared not show in public. American cigarettes were a premium.

"It is awful hard for me," Lionel said. "I try to remember just a little, but my head is like a sieve. Everything falls out. I can hardly understand a word, much less memorize it all."

"Lionel, it will come. Tonight you and I will review the leg and then we'll go over the biochemistry, which I think I can manage to understand."

Supper was always the same for me—a hamburger patty grilled on my hot plate, some cheese, lots of bread and a cup of Nescafe. I wanted some fresh vegetables, especially a tomato, but we had been sternly warned that tomatoes were a common source of TB. This illness was the scourge of the medical students in Toulouse.

The hotel smelled like a cheap, greasy diner at dinner time. Lionel and I worked until eleven, but it became quickly and unhappily apparent to me that Lionel was simply not going to learn the voluminous material. He had been away from school for too long. His concentration was earnest, but ineffective. He looked so tired when he left my room that it broke my heart. His eyes, swollen and red, were set far back in his drained face, and he barely had the strength or will to speak. Everything had become a huge effort.

I made a schedule for myself to memorize and draw each section, a schedule corresponding to that of the professor.

At the stroke of midnight, there was a gentle knock on the door. Monique was standing there, dangling an unlit cigarette in her wondrously feminine hand.

"I have come to help you. You are not too tired?"

"I have been hoping you would come. I was going to knock on your door if you didn't."

Monique lived two rooms down the corridor. The shutters of her room were always tightly shut, but soft music came through the door, as did hints of her intoxicating perfume.

All over the bed and the chairs and the entire room I sprinkled Old Spice after-shave lotion, hoping to get rid of the ever-present smell of formaldehyde—or at least to blunt some of its sharpness.

She wore a different dress and blouse and high heels, which made her shapely legs even more exciting.

We sat by the desk, she moving her delicate fingers over the page, translating the complicated language of medicine, occasionally pausing to turn her seductive brown eyes towards me with a smile, which only served to make her even more alluring. By one in the morning I could no longer restrain myself, and I kissed her cheek gently.

"*Mais,* no. You have to study, *Cheri,*" she reprimanded. "You are a poor student, aren't you? Not like the others?"

"Yes, but why do you ask?"

"*Comme ca,* like that."

She rose and disappeared again. I began to wonder if I hadn't really invented her. She appeared only at or shortly after midnight. For weeks after she had left, I stole past her room every night, using my trip to the common toilet as a pretext. No sound came from the room, no light from under her door. Sometimes I knocked softly, knowing full well that the echo carried throughout the court. It was like announcing that I was in insatiable heat.

Studying was becoming more and more difficult; also, now I devoted more of my efforts to Lionel. We cooked together on his little stove, or, rather, I should say that he cooked all sorts of concoctions with sausages and lots of bread. Lionel began to change noticeably as the days passed into weeks, and the changes did not augur well. He couldn't remember the day of the week before stressful lessons, especially those dealing with the anatomy of the brain and all its highly complicated tracts and connections. I was managing, barely. I found the heart to be the most exciting organ, especially the marvelously intricate functional anatomy—or was it because I was a hopeless romantic?

"'The seat of the soul resides in the heart,' according to Aristotle," I said to him one night.

He laughed wearily and said, "That's not what the Bible says. God resides in all of man, in all of us, even we negroes."

He had a small radio in his room, an ancient Zenith, and he listened to the Armed Forces station that played American jazz. When Louis Armstrong sang, he sang along with him—"I'll get by, as long as I have you..." and he did a little tap dance to the music, trying to rouse himself. But he was so lonely and frustrated that tears came to his eyes. He was a shy and humble man who could have had many friends, but he had convinced himself that white folks truly didn't care for the likes of him. He wasn't wrong. The French were, outwardly, very tolerant to the blacks. Lionel found this amusing. He knew better. I could see the pain in his eyes when one of the students would casually ask him to turn his hand over so he could see if it was white on the surface of the palm. The students knew of the vicious attacks against the blacks in the South and knew all about the lynchings. They did make an extra effort to be kind, but it was cruelly condescending. They regarded blacks as poor, child-like victims.

One night, at the end of November, Lionel invited me to dine with him in one of the marvelous restaurants.

"You know, it's Thanksgiving. We will have our own Thanksgiving here."

We found a small bistro on the Rue de Bourg, and for five dollars we could ill afford we had a delicious six-course meal. To keep some semblance of Thanksgiving tradition, we ordered *coc au vin*, the closest thing we could find on the menu to turkey. We drank a cheap Algerian wine. By the end of the dinner, we had both grown mellow and melancholy.

"You really miss your young lady," he said. "I see the sadness in your eyes. Man, you are young and good-looking. You will find dozens of others. It's a sure thing."

"Lionel, I know, but one needs time and some money."

Monique had disappeared out of my life. Embarrassment—or was it plain shyness?—prevented me from making any inquiries about her. I felt offended, hurt. My ego was shattered. I concluded that I just wasn't good enough for her. But the memory lingered.

*

In the weeks that followed, I could study little and waited for the night to come, hoping that there would soon be that gentle knock on my door which would relieve me of my misery, lift the weight of depression from me.

By the beginning of December I decided to get out a bit. There was a student restaurant which I decided to try. It was cold and raining, and I took the long walk to the medieval building through the dark, narrow streets of Toulouse. A pungent odor surrounded me from the sewage that flowed in the gutters.

The restaurant was crowded with French and Algerian students, all waiting in line with iron trays. I followed the line and took one of the unappetizing metal trays, along with a glass and worn silverware. Military style, they filled each section of the plate with french fries, sausages and withered tomatoes, and filled the glass with Algerian table wine. At the cashiers I had to present an identity card, which I had never bothered to get at the bursar's office. Standing directly in back of me was a tall, scrawny-looking black woman holding her tray, stacked with double portions of vegetables, meat, and two glasses of wine.

"Oh, he is American. Let him go by. I will explain everything to him," she said in French.

"*Merci*," I said, grateful for her concern and kindness.

"Don't waste your time in French. I'm an American. Follow me and I will teach you the ropes."

There were miles of long wooden tables in this cafeteria, with the haggard and exhausted students eating from their metal plates. The smells of food permeated the air, mixed with smoke—such dense smoke—and wine and unwashed bodies and clothes. There wasn't another American in sight, except for my new friend, Clarice.

She found her own spot and thrust her thin body on the bench, between two other students.

"If you don't push and shove, these frogs won't let you in," she said simply.

The scene looked like a movie I once saw, one starring George Raft at Alcatraz.

"So you came to join the Foreign Legion in Toulouse. You look like a bright kid. Why aren't you in Yale or some other spiffy joint?"

I didn't answer her.

"How long have you been here?" I asked instead.

"Five years," she said, "and I will stay until I pass my exams."

The French system of medical school consists of a five to six-year course. Two examinations are given, one at the end of two years, and then the final at the termination of the studies. The examination period itself takes months, involving ten to twelve exams. Students must get a passing grade in eighteen of the twenty exams. Otherwise, they have to repeat all the exams the following year. Some students take ten years or more to pass their exams. Some give up. Some simply get too old to care.

"This is a good place to learn French," she said, "but you need a girlfriend to really learn the language. Do you have any money?"

"No."

"Too bad. That will make it very hard. With money you get slides, a good skeleton, good English texts and even tutors. And, of course, you need money to take a woman for coffee."

"Do you have money?" I asked her.

"*C'est drol,* that is funny. Would I be eating in this prison cafeteria? I manage."

She wore a long nondescript dress. Her hair was unkempt, she looked shabby, but she burst with life and enthusiasm. Most of the students who passed us greeted her. I must have met a dozen students in only a few minutes.

"Come home with me. I have a roommate you may like. She speaks no English, but you aren't a bad-looking guy."

We finished eating and left the cafeteria. We walked with long quick strides through the windy streets for almost an hour; then we reached a row of small houses.

"We live on the ground floor—two bedrooms, a kitchen, a small living room."

"Danielle!" she yelled. "We have a visitor!"

Everywhere in the room were books and papers, most opened, strewn on the floor and on the kitchen table.

"I will make some coffee," she said. "Push them aside and find a spot. I usually sit on the floor."

She continued speaking while she made the coffee, but I was unable to hear a word.

Danielle came into the room wearing a housecoat. The light in the room was dim, but I could see she had dark hair and was buxom, with large round eyes. She was not a particularly attractive woman, and she appeared considerably older than I.

"There you are, Danielle. Were you sleeping? This is our new friend, an American medical student. He has to learn French because he will never pass."

"*Enchante,*" she said.

We all sat on the floor drinking coffee, while Clarice chatted on, and then she suddenly rose and said, "I have to study and leave you two alone. Before you leave—when you leave—you can borrow my bones. I have a very good skull, femur, radius, pelvis, and hand. The rest you will have to scrounge around for. You have to learn each crease on the bones and holes in the skull and what goes through them. If you pass anatomy you are on your way. Most of the students flunk anatomy and biochemistry the first time around. Hope you do better."

To carry on a conversation with a total stranger without knowing the language is not without its difficulties. Danielle was able to follow some of my English, and we limped along. It grew late. Classes began at eight in the morning, and I wondered how I would get back.

There were no buses. Clarice solved my dilemma when she rejoined us.

"It's too late to go back to your hotel," she said. She must have read my thoughts. "Stay here and we can leave together in the morning. You can sleep with Danielle. She won't mind."

Clarice explained to Danielle, who simply said, "*D'accord,*" All right.

Danielle's room was neat and organized. There was a cross on the wall and a wonderful painting of the Virgin Mary on her dresser. No books or magazines cluttered up her room. The night was chilly, and I was glad to be under the covers of the large down feather duvet. Soon she was beside me, while her robe was neatly folded over the chair.

It was good not to be alone, but all night I thought of Monique, even as we made love.

In the morning she served me *café au lait* in a large cup, and a croissant, while I was still in bed.

Clarice yelled from the other room, "Get the hell out of bed. I never go to class before noon. I am only doing this for you. We have to catch the bus at the place Essquarole to make the first lecture."

By the look Danielle gave me as I left, I knew she understood I would not return.

*

In Toulouse, the week or so before Christmas, there were no signs that the holiday was fast approaching. Few decorations bedecked the stores; occasionally, a Christmas tree was visible. Christmas in France was a serious, somber religious holiday. After midnight, after church, all the restaurants and homes had a huge dinner, called le Reunion. The Americans almost always took this time to go skiing or traveling so the hotel was almost empty. The concierge, Madame Lelang, was a kind woman and she had a large decorated tree in her living room.

"Monsieur is staying here for the holidays?"

"Yes, it is better. It will give me a chance to do more studying."

She knew I was lying, because I was late by a week or two with the rent. I was staying in Toulouse because I was broke.

"Well, then, you must join us, if you have the time, of course."

Lionel cooked a small goose and sweet potatoes on his stove, and we listened to the Armed Forces network program that played Christmas carols all night. We drank champagne and wine and sang along. Christmas in Toulouse was hardly Christmas in Vermont.

After midnight, I staggered back to my room and fell asleep on my bed. I didn't hear the knock on the door, but felt a gentle kiss on my cheek and knew I was dreaming again. Monique stood above me, perfumed, lovely in a red dress. Only the light filtering in from the hall entered the small room.

"Merry Christmas, *cheri*," she said, and handed me a Christmas card and a large chocolate heart. But it was no dream when I pulled her towards me. I needed her to be real, genuine, nourishing. She was.

*

In the morning, without makeup, she looked even more beautiful than the night before.

"Where have you been all these months? I waited and waited, disturbed and even annoyed. If you had only written or called me!"

"Well, you know. It was better this way. My father was ill, and I had to stay in the country with my parents. Let's be happy," she said, "and we must begin Christmas Day the French way."

She returned a few minutes later with a bottle of champagne, two glasses, real coffee, two croissants, and a small radio.

"We better stay home today. It is snowing too much."

In our rooms, night and day were one. Monique brought two blue candles, a miniature Christmas tree, a plastic reindeer in a glass, and a beautiful doll with brown hair. She owned a small turntable and a collection of Edith Piaf, Charles Trenet, Yves Montand, and Frank Sinatra. She transformed this small depressing room into a magic wonderland. It became night again. The flickering light of the candle reflected in the mirror of the armoire and made her silken skin glow with a maddening intensity.

We laughed and made love and slept, and ate delicious French cheeses, and drank more wine, and smoked Phillip Morris cigarettes.

When I felt hungry she made an omelette of herbs. We ate chocolate and bread in bed. Sometimes my eyes wandered to the section
on the ceiling where I had a blackboard mounted with biochemistry
formulas. I strained to read the formulas in the candlelight. Monique
made haste to prevent me from returning to reality by placing her
small delicate hands over my eyes.

"*Mon petite chou*, there is time enough for your chemistry on the
ceiling. There is enough here. *Fait le pratique sur mois*, practice on me."

We whispered like lovers, told of everything in our hearts while
listening, enraptured, to Edith Piaf singing, "*Mon Amour.*"

"From now on we speak only in French," she said, "and if you
don't understand, *tampi*, too bad, your loss. You must learn French very
well because otherwise you won't pass your exams."

An entire day and another night went by, and in the morning she
left the room with all her lovely possessions, except for the doll with
the brown hair.

"In case you forget about me, or you have another girlfriend, my
poupee will remind you. See how her large brown eyes stare at you.
Beware, *mon amour!*"

*

I must confess that I had completely forgotten about Lionel, who
must have surmised why I hadn't surfaced for two days. I knocked on
his door and was surprised that he was not at his desk. He kept his
room immaculate. He used a pine spray in the room, lest there was
the slightest chance of offending the cleaning lady. All our rooms were
malodorous, reeking, but not his. His bed was made, the towels neatly
folded, and there was nothing in the room except for his cooking utensils
and some cans of food, neatly stacked, a bottle of wine, and a carton
of Phillip Morris. His clothing was gone, and there was a note on the
desk, and a large envelope addressed to me.

Dear Lover Boy,

*I did not want to disturb you, but I have to leave. I am too lonely and it is no use. I
can't ever learn all of this stuff. I tried as you well know. I don't belong in medical
school and will make out fine at home. You will be a great doctor someday, and I
want to thank you for being so kind to an old man. Please take my oil cooker and*

food, and radio. The envelope is for you. When you get your M.D. and make good money, you can repay me. What use are French francs to me anyway? Take care of yourself. Peace and love.

Inside the envelope there was thirty thousand francs—about five hundred dollars!—enough money for me to finish off the year in luxury and to buy that needed skeleton.

My throat was dry, my eyes moist. Dear kind Lionel, my irreplaceable friend.

*

Monique had disappeared again for two days, and when she returned late at night, she brought a little present, a "good luck pen."

"I didn't come to see you because you must study. It is very difficult to pass the exams here in France, you know, and I want to stay here with you, but if you do not succeed, I will be to blame."

"And if you don't come here, I will also fail because I cannot concentrate enough to study. So it is better you are here, and I will study like a mad fool, drawing energy from you." A smile and a pause. "Where do you disappear to? You are so mysterious."

"*Mon cheri,* mystery and longing is the secret of lasting love, so we say in French."

"Where do you go?" I asked her again.

"Oh, you know, I have parents I must stay with in the country, outside of Toulouse. We live in a vineyard, and my father makes wine. Someday we will perhaps go together?"

*

On weekends, Monique became more generous with her time. Knowing we would soon see each other was the motivation I needed to work twice as hard and efficiently. We met often in the center of town, at the *Place Capitale,* in the *Cafés des Artistes,* where, apparently, Toulouse Lautrec had once come to do some paintings.

"It is better that those nosy people in the hotel don't see us together," she said. "*Je suis tres propre,* I am very morale, you know. In France, we keep our private lives very discreet."

It became apparent that Monique was no ordinary shop girl. She was educated, *au courant*, as the French say. She always looked as if she had just walked out of a stylish dress shop. Scarves of colorful silk were as much a part of her as her beautiful brown hair. She was wearing a leather coat, a blue and brown scarf casually around her neck. It was becoming cold, and inside the cafe there was the smell of warm wine and cigarettes. She was sitting demurely by a small round table near the window. The late afternoon light made her beautiful hair shimmer. She was sipping on a cup of coffee, and just for a moment I wanted to look at her as from a distance, objectively. Her small lips were on the porcelain rim of the cup; one of her adorable fingers with the red polish rested on her chin; her legs were tightly crossed, her ankles touching. She must have just arrived because her cheeks were fresh and red as apples from the cold December air.

When I approached her, her face lit up, and she said, "*Tien, tien, mon petite chou*. Did you work well?"

"Very well. So well I have the day free."

"And the night?"

"Of course, the night."

She gave me a tiny kiss on my cheek, and her eyes glowed with such love and passion that I wanted to smother her with kisses right then and there.

"What would you like today?" she asked.

"Are you serious? You need to ask?"

"My hungry, starving student. Good things are better if you have to wait a little for them, you know."

"I know, I know, only too well. I've waited a lot. Would you mind coming along with me. I have to buy a skeleton."

"*Mon Dieu*, he has gone crazy. I am not good enough for you. You need another one with no flesh."

We took the tram to the Rue de Metz, to one of the students' homes. He was an Algerian living in a small attic in a huge and ancient mansion. His room looked not unlike mine, and smelled as bad. When he saw Monique his eyes nearly popped from their sockets.

He wanted seventy dollars for the skeleton.

Monique whispered to me in English, "Oh, no. That is too much for old bones. Tell him you have only forty dollars."

Right at that moment a bitter war was being fought in North Africa, the French Foreign Legion trying to subdue a revolt of the

Algerians who demanded their independence.

Monique was right. He accepted forty dollars.

We put the skeleton in small shopping bags, and Monique carried the skull, which wouldn't fit.

"Is it a boy or girl?" she asked. "How can you tell?"

"If it starts rattling when you touch it, it is a boy," I said. "This is a girl. You can tell by the pelvis."

"Oh, voila, then I have to be a little jealous when you are alone at night with this slender mademoiselle."

We took the tram, staying close, our bodies touching as we held the skeleton. The French are *blasé*—or is it jaded?— even the bare head in her arms caused no stir. Part of the skeleton leg protruded from the bag, and this was accepted, too, but when the tram made a sudden halt and all the bones came flying out of the bag, it was simply too much, even for the French. The passengers gasped at the parts of the skeleton strewn all over the floor. It looked like children about to play pick up sticks.

We quickly gathered the bones and got off the tram.

"Oh, he is a medical student," someone yelled, and they all laughed and envied us the way we looked at each other.

Love makes you feel confident, unafraid. It gives you the inner strength and security to make fun of everything, and makes you want to laugh at that which once seemed so terribly serious. Love gave me a sense of freedom I had never known. I could breathe again, drawing in huge and delicious gulps of clean air.

*

Now we were together most of the time. While I struggled nightly with the difficult task of learning, Monique stayed in my room. Languidly dozing on the bed or reading a book of poetry, she would catch my eye and wave to me as if she were in a distant field. Sometimes, she stole behind me and touched my head with her lips while her arms encircled my drooping shoulders. Slowly, I would turn my head and her face would be near mine. I followed the curve of her thin eyebrows and touched her small, curved nose, until the tip of my finger ran along her lips.

"Not yet, *mon dieu*. Go back to your histology. There are only a few months left."

*

Like most of the other students, I stopped attending classes because there was just not enough time to do everything. The day began at five in the morning, Monique sleeping soundly while I brewed some Nescafe. Fatigue was one feeling I never felt now. So inspired, so driven was I, that grueling hours of study even became enjoyable. Learning is not usually fun, but I had my own private drive. Everything was fun. Carnal pleasures and scholarly endeavors coexisted, each prompting and enhancing the other.

I was one of the lucky few, the recipient of those two treasured civilized gifts. When each cell of my brain was filled, overcharged, each synapse worn to the ground, Monique knew at once by my drooping eyes and planned a brief change to allow my brain to rest.

*

We took the train to visit the ruins in Arles, the old museums and buildings in Montepellier, and on one weekend we took the train to the Riviera.

Nice in the month of March was cold and windy. This great playground of the world now belonged to the people who made their home by the sea. The empty cafes looked like ghosts, and the hotels, even the famous Negresco, were stark and awesome—a grand lady asleep, without makeup, but still elegant and beautiful.

The stony beach which soon would be covered with beautiful people was now washed by the sea. The salt air cleared my brain. In just a few hours I was reborn, anxious to return to the job. Such wisdom in such a young woman. It was as if she herself had once endured the rigors of being a medical student.

As the days to the exams grew nearer, I became more nervous, even neurotic. In the middle of our lovemaking, I would jump up from the bed to check on something I thought I had forgotten.

"*Mon dieu,* of all the men in the world, I have to fall in love with a medical student," she said. Physical pleasures could not scotch my fears and anxiety. Nothing that Monique said or did could erase the accelerating madness in my brain, filled to overflowing with images of dancing arteries and nerve connections and complex and intricate formulas. My texts and I merged into one—a necessary but loveless marriage.

Now, in the final weeks, I saw Monique only once or twice a week.

*

Spring arrived, and the air was so fresh and gentle, the cafes were again alive, majestically lining the streets filled with young lovers. Late at night, when Monique was not with me, I would take a break from my studies and walk through the old narrow streets of centuries-old houses. The streets were charming, but many had a stench from the open sewers running through them. I would recite out loud whatever I had memorized that day. Onlookers simply took me for a madman. They nodded and moved on.

Prostitutes of all sizes and shapes, young and old, stood along these dark streets calling "*Vien, cheri,* a little love in the night," which I found amusing. This was part of the charm of Toulouse.

Some of the faces looked familiar to me because they were required by law to check in the clinic each week to be tested for venereal diseases.

Their carte *d'identitá* had to be signed stating they were free of disease otherwise they would be arrested by the police.

The medical students were assigned to their care which was part of the clinical training.

The final exams were like a lottery. Two subjects are picked from a hat, and these become the written portion. If a passing grade was achieved, then the student was eligible to take the oral examinations.

On the morning of the lottery the students gathered in the medieval courtyard of the medical school. It was a lovely morning, and there was a carnival atmosphere. The younger students, those who did not flunk the examinations the first time around, were kicking a soccer ball, others were smoking furiously pacing back and forth still high from the Maxidol they took the night before to cram for the examinations. Monique and I stood in the shadows of the old pillars of courtyard. She looked elegant and beautiful, her arm around me, my heart racing. Would I pass? It was impossible to know all the subjects in detail, especially the anatomy. Each student hoped painstakingly that the two subjects picked would be their strongest. My hopes focused on anatomy and biochemistry, or physiology.

One of the proctors, Bernard Bouley from the anatomy laboratory, was standing in the center of the circle of students, holding the traditional worn top hat containing white slips of paper, upon which, written in gold, were the names of each subject.

Outside of the circle, Monique pushed closer to my side, waiting for the chosen student to put a hand into the hat. A blond-haired student that I had never seen stepped smartly forward. He was apparently quite a popular man because they all shouted *"Alle, Alle,* Jean Paul, go, go, Jean Paul."

"You don't know him?" Monique asked. "He is very well liked. He was picked the king of the medical school ball this year."

I knew of the ball, but I hadn't had the money or the clothes to attend. Also, I didn't really care very much.

"It is histology and legal medicine," the blond boy shouted. Some of the students groaned with pain while others cheered. I was absolutely crestfallen because these were the subjects I had studied the least.

"Don't look so doomed," Monique said. "You have some weeks more before the exam and you can make a quick review, *n'est-ce pas?*"

*

The next three weeks were like a nightmare. I saw little of Monique.

"We must not drain any energy from you," she said. "I have a little present for you to make your brain better." She gave me a handful of vials with a green solution inside. It looked like something to put into a bath to make bubbles.

"It is glutamic acid. All the students use it. It makes you calm and helps you to memorize better."

Pharmacology was one of the subjects I studied, and I panicked. Had I already forgotten what I learned? I knew it was an amino acid, but I could not find it in the text. In one of the lectures the professor had mentioned it briefly. When she left I threw the vials in the wastebasket in frustration.

The Hotel Henri became one large study hall. None of us slept very much. We crammed desperately, trying to digest everything written in our voluminous textbook. We formed small study groups with Rosenberg, Ralph and an Algerian student, and studied questions handed down by students who have gone before us. We had to know every crease on the bones of the body and skull, every formula, all the

French laws pertaining to legal medical aspects of murder and geno-
cide, euthanasia, homosexuality, perversion and drug abuse.

We were reviewing and mumbling to ourselves like a group of Jesuits
reading their breviary in a monastery. Even those lucky few students
who had superior memories had to keep their noses close to the grind-
stone. Our task was made even more difficult because, of course, it all
had to be learned in French.

Some of the students relied on Maxidol, a drug which allowed
them to stay awake and study all night.

During those grueling nights and days, Monique weaved in and
out of the room, staying just long enough to be embraced. Most of
the time I hardly noticed her, but her perfume filled the room; or she
left some bread and cheese, or a paté or sausages or chocolates. My
underclothes and socks were cleaned and folded neatly on the bed, and
she left little notes: "*Mon petite chou*, work hard, I miss you."

*

The night before the examination the silence of the hotel was broken
by dozens of young voices, shouting women speaking in English and
laughing. Bearded, in my pajamas, I slipped out of my tiny room, and
saw dozens of beautiful young women checking in and rushing up the
narrow stairs to their rooms. Holiday On Ice, a British Ice Capades
group, had checked into the hotel and were friendly and anxious to
spend the evening with us. When I returned to my room expecting
to see Monique, I saw instead a cute young blond sitting on my bed.
She tried to entice me. Monique was so much more attractive and
womanly. It took a lot of cajoling to have her leave.

"Are you one of those funny chaps," she asked me.

"No, just in love with someone else and I have a examination to
take in a few hours," I told her.

For the rest of the night there was laughter and singing throughout
the hotel.

Sleep was impossible. It was nerve wracking to have this last
important night sabotaged by the Ice Capades ladies.

*

Our group arrived at the examination hall bleary eyed and fearful. It was a written examination for both subjects and it was a miracle how sharp my brain functioned in spite of the raucous, sleepless, night before.

By the middle of May, it was over. Euphoria mixed with silent prayers and more sleepless nights while I waited for the results to be posted on the bulletin board of the medical school.

If I flunked, I half convinced myself that it mattered little to me as long as Monique was with me. This rationalization offered some relief from the strain. The word was out in the cafe at Place Capitale that the names of the successful candidates had been posted that morning. We rushed, like the insane, to the bulletin board, Monique holding and squeezing my icy hand. Some students came back cheering, others bemoaning fate—another year of torture.

Rosenberg came back smiling, and so did Ralph. Monique insisted that she look at the bulletin board.

"I will bring you good luck, my dearest."

I watched her trim body stretching to see the names, and she returned a few minutes later, silently, with not a trace of expression on her face.

"*Eh bien, mon doctor,* you passed!" she squealed and flung her arms around me and wouldn't stop kissing my teary eyes. We jumped and danced, squeezed until our ribs hurt.

Although it was only the first year, it was the essential test, even though the many years ahead would be as trying as this one. If I knew then what lay ahead of me, I doubt that I would have continued.

My euphoria was quickly dampened when I received a letter from the Board of Examiners in New York, signed by the commissioner of education (who would, in a few years, be removed from office for improper conduct).

Unfortunately, the state of New York Board of Examiners stated, a degree from a Toulouse medical school would no longer be acceptable in the U.S. I had to transfer to a medical school in Switzerland if my degree was to be transferable. Money had by now run out, and I would have to return to New York to work during the summer as a waiter in a summer resort in the Catskills. But none of that truly perturbed or disheartened me—except having to leave Monique.

Now, school over, we spent every precious moment together.

Everyone should be in love at least once in the spring. Old

Toulouse became a garden of love. Miles of opened cafés packed with young and old, sitting, talking, eating, thinking, in the young sun of the new day. Women in large aprons scrubbed the sidewalks in front of their homes. The outside markets, a kaleidoscope of colorful tulips and daffodils, intermingled with the displays of hundreds of cheeses, sausages, breads, meats, and fish. Everywhere were the smells and whispers of spring. It was intoxicating.

Monique and I were like hundreds of others, holding hands, bending our heads together, always kissing each other, sharing those wonderful sweet secrets and glances only lovers know. And the laughter, which was as much a part of love as hugging, whispering and the endearing naughty and absolutely carnal thoughts.

My French was fluent now, thanks to Monique, and we rarely spoke in English. French was meant for making love; it is more romantic than any other language.

"I want to know everything about you," I told her, "what you looked like when you were a child, your family, all your secret thoughts and fantasies; yes, even about all your lovers."

"*Mon dieu*, this is too much. A French woman never speaks of her old lovers. You want to possess me like a *poupee*, like my doll. You let me keep a little of myself, young doctor-to-be."

We were sitting on the concrete parapet facing the river, the Haute Garronee, that snakes through the burgundy country and down to the region of France, called the Midi. Men and women were there by the hundreds, their fishing poles in hand.

"I am jealous of your dreams," I told her. "Each smile you give to someone else is a loss for me."

"*Arrete, mon petit folle,* stop my little fool. That you have so little experience with women is obvious. Of course we love each other today, it is spring. But tomorrow, when the bloom is off the rose, who knows? When you return to New York you may come back married."

"Never, you are the first love I have ever known, and I don't want anyone else. You'll see. Wait for me."

*

I wrote to Monique every night from New York. She was with me every minute in spirit. She answered in her delicate handwriting. I tried to contact Lionel, but he was no longer living at the address he gave me. All my letters were returned: "address unknown."

I worked as a waiter at a hotel in the Catskill Mountains, and the summer passed. I was the classic obsequious waiter but it did not earn me more tips.

"A medical student, everyone in the Catskills is a medical student," one miserable guest at the Napanach Country Club said to forewarn me that no larger tip was coming for having that distinction. I had earned just enough money to squeeze through the coming year. I had wanted to earn more so I could take Monique to Nice and buy her fancy gifts.

October finally arrived. I had survived the misery of the summer knowing soon I would return to the country I learned to love and to Monique. I missed "everything that flows in Paris" as Jean-Paul Sartre wrote. The smells and sounds and colors of Toulouse were with me each moment of the day. At least once a week a letter had arrived from Monique, but in the two weeks before I was preparing to leave for France, none arrived. Not hearing from her was agony.

*

Returning to Europe was not an easy journey to make. Plane fare was very expensive and the Atlantic crossing by ship took five to six days.

In October, the sea becomes rough and exciting. I paced the decks like a wild caged animal as the winds howled, bent and raised this 44,500 ton ship as if she were a canoe. Soon, I would be seeing Monique, and neither a storm nor any power on earth was going to stop me. The II de France made it safely home, and I disembarked filled with excitement and impatience. First, there was the train from Le Harvre to Paris, and then another train, the night train, the Oriental Express, to Toulouse.

At six in the morning I arrived in Toulouse. The taxi driver was a typical Toulousian, wearing a beret and singing his words. It felt good to converse in French again. The streets were empty, gray, sad-looking, and when we arrived at the Hotel Henri, there was one light on over the sign that read "Tourisme." My mouth was dry and I felt my heart pounding through my shirt.

Monsieur Lelang greeted me affectionately at the desk. He looked like he had just climbed out of his bed. Nothing had changed over the last few months. The straw chairs, the small center table, and the posters advertising the ski resorts in the Pyrennes on the side yellow wall were all in their same places.

My eyes rested on the narrow circular stairs that led to the second floor, where once I lived in my room of paradise. "Does Monique have the same room?" I asked.

"No, she is no longer here, Monsieur."

A sledgehammer hit my head.

"Where did she go?" I asked in panic. "Did she not leave a message? She knew when I was to arrive. I wrote her a dozen times."

"She was picked up by the police," he said quietly.

"The police? Monique? Are you sure? Why? What happened?"

"Eh bien, she did not go for a check-up and failed to register!"

"Check up? What are you saying?"

"In France, all the *putaines* have to register, and a doctor exams them once a month."

"*Putaine?* Monique a prostitute? Not possible. Are you mad?"

"Everyone knew it," Madame Lelang said. "We were sure you did. We had warned her not to bother you, and we threatened to make her leave the hotel."

Madame Lelang saw my face, pale and perspiring, almost lifeless.

"Please sit, Monsieur. We really did not know you were not informed. She never told you, or asked you for money?"

"Of course not. She brought me presents. I never gave her anything. She said she visited her parents' vineyards, not far from here, when she was away."

"My poor man, you were so deceived," Madam Lelang said.

"I have to find her. I must see her. It is surely a mistake."

But it was not a mistake. The police had her registered as a whore, a call girl. After her mandatory medical check-up for venereal disease, she paid a small fine, was released and had not been seen again. That is why she had disappeared so suddenly. Everything she told me was a lie. She never once even hinted at her profession, and I had never seen her at the hospital clinic. Perhaps that was why she made love so magnificently—an artist at her craft. Does she tell such lies to all her customers? I really believed she loved me. Sometimes I wondered what she found so wonderful about a poor medical student when she was so beautiful and alluring.

I turned away from the desk because I felt sick, my stomach knotted. I was dead inside. Another part of my life was over. When I boarded the train again several hours later for Switzerland, I thought, for an instant, that I saw her in her leather coat, a colorful scarf flying in the breeze, walking arm in arm with a man with gray hair, leaving the station.

Scarlet Fever

I GOT A JOB selling women's undergarments. Mr. White had a tiny store on 8th Avenue and 48th Street with a few shelves of bras and panties. But when women came in and saw a teenage boy behind the counter they walked out.

Mr. White was a white-haired man with the largest eyebrows I had ever seen. He was a pleasant Irishman who kept telling me to be patient and work hard.

And I did, standing for three hours after school trying to sell panties.

*

The school year ended and another hot summer was waiting for me with nothing to do. When Mr. White learned I had no plans he proposed I work on his farm in the country, taking care of his dog and the chickens, and mowing the grass.

He drove me along Route 27 to his farmhouse in Saugerties, New York. The house was a standard two-story clapboard home, with the farm in back. He gave me a nice bedroom upstairs.

The chicken coup had a hundred chickens. My job was to collect the eggs and examine them with a candle. If any had spots I was instructed to throw them away. The chickens were lying on the eggs and I had to pick them up and run my hand underneath their warm bodies. It was a battle each time, as the chickens pecked my hand. I finally found some gloves and the egg picking was no longer painful. But from then on I was no longer fond of chicken dinners or salads.

After picking the eggs and cleaning the waste and placing water in all the troughs, I took Mr. White's German Shepherd for a walk. This was my favorite part of the day and we became great friends, as the dog reminded me of my dog, Astor, in Danzig. Astor protected me from the German kids who were taught to hate Jews and who when given the chance, tried to beat me up.

*

One morning I was walking the dog along the road leading to town when a tall, nice-looking man came to greet me. He asked me who I was and I said I worked on the farm for Mr. White.

The nice-looking man invited me to his home for dinner. Chicken, of course.

The following weekend Mr. White came with a young, beautiful woman to clean.

I helped her wash the windows. She wore a low-cut blouse exposing her breasts every time she bent down. She smiled and I ran away, not wanting her to see the sudden bulge in my pants.

The next weekend I wanted to be ready for her arrival, so I could help her clean the windows. But that meant I had to finish my own chores first. In my haste I forgot to turn the water off and the troughs overflowed. Some of the chickens were on the ground, beating their wings in the shallow water.

I panicked and worked like a comet, wiping up the wet coup the best I could, hoping the hot summer day would dry them.

I was mowing the front lawn when the black Ford station wagon arrived with Mr. White and the young, beautiful woman.

Mr. White immediately went to inspect the chicken coup. He ran back into the house, asking why everything was wet and the chickens looked sick.

I confessed what happened. The following morning most of them had died of polio.

Mr. White didn't give me a ride back to Manhattan this time but put me on the bus with a disappointed scowl. "Don't pick farming as a profession," he advised me. "Try medicine."

*

A few weeks later I started to have a terrible sore throat with fever and vomiting. My parents were worried I might have polio. I hadn't even told them about the chickens, and I wondered if I could have caught it from them. But the doctor diagnosed me with scarlet fever.

I developed a red rash all over my body. Scarlet fever was a very serious ailment. Often children developed heart disease as a result, and many died.

I was ordered to bed for three weeks and the health department made it mandatory to keep me in isolation. They placed a plaque on the our front door:

BEWARE ISOLATION! NO ENTRANCE PERMITTED!

This was routine for cases of scarlet fever. A tall ugly nurse came each morning. She looked like one of the German Nazi nurses who had been so cruel to me when I had been taken to a hospital in Berlin many years before. But instead of wearing a starched white uniform she was dressed in a blue uniform with yellow buttons and carried a large leather bag.

The floors of the apartment had to be scrubbed with Lysol. There were no antibiotics, except for sulfur used by the military. Dr. Rosenblatt came each day to listen to my heart and lungs.

I had been even more sick in Danzig, when my parents took me to see a famous doctor in Berlin, who diagnosed me to have brucellosis. At that time the Kras had been very rich and my parents could afford the best care.

Now I experienced the fateful combination of poverty and illness. Where was our rich cousin who took us to the Waldorf but soon after dropped us like strangers?

*

After my isolation ended my mother arranged to send me to a convalescent home for poor children. We took the subway to Coney Island, a long trip. Sitting across was a young girl with curly hair who kept staring at me, maybe with pity. I must have looked half dead.

She was so beautiful I could not help staring back. I wanted to think we both fell in love at that moment. I certainly did. But maybe I was delusional from my illness and isolation. I didn't want to get off the train, to part with her, knowing I would never see her again. I remember her to this day.

My mother led me from the station toward the beach, where there was a big white house surrounded by a fence. The gate was open and we climbed up the stairs to the foyer, where Mother spoke to the receptionist.

I was escorted to a ward with twenty beds lined up in a row. I was given the first one, by the door. I felt miserable, abandoned, alone. My mother had given me some candies, which I hid under my pillow. The other boys in the ward, mostly pale and thin, and around the same age, didn't return my greetings or pay me much attention.

The next morning I felt weak and hungry. I could barely climb the stairs to the dining room.

Each boy had to have a tall glass of warm milk each day and we were ordered to drink it, skin and all. A fat nun in a long white dress with a huge cross dangling between her breasts looked at me as she ladled my milk from a large pot and said with a scowl, "Oh, you're that refugee Jew boy."

I hated warm milk. I wanted to vomit as I saw the large skin floating on top. I went to the bathroom, adjacent to the dining room, and spilled the milk into the toilet.

I returned to the dining room and lined up for cereal and eggs, which I ate in record time.

Afterward the counselor took us out to the playground to play baseball, a game I had never played. I sat on the bench and watched the other boys bat. When my turn came I didn't know how to hold it. I swung it wildly, stumbling over the plate, and the ball almost hit me in the head. I couldn't wait to return to the bench.

The counselor said, "You're going to have to learn how to play baseball. We play baseball in America."

The next sport was boxing, and that was a game I knew, having been taught by the sea captain who plotted our escape from Danzig. The counselor put the gloves on my hands and told me how to hold them, which I already knew, and explained we would fight for three rounds.

At first I was battered by my older opponent. But I didn't cry. Instead I got angry and began to pound the blond-haired kid until blood came from his nose and the counselor stopped the fight.

*

I could not stand the place and decided I must escape. While we were taking our afternoon nap one day I snuck out to the beach and wrote HELP HELP HELP on the sand, then returned to the ward before anyone knew I was missing.

But how was anyone supposed to rescue me? How would they know who had written the message? So the following day I became bolder and decided to take the subway home.

But I had no money.

The counselor was waiting for me when I got back.

"You're healthy enough to run away," the counselor said. "Do you want me to call your mother and have her pick you up?"

*

I hung around the neighborhood, still feeling washed out. One day I wandered onto 98th Street and saw a nice-looking girl. I spoke to her and we became friends. Her name was Florence. I wrote her a letter and told her I loved her. I placed the letter in my woolen robe.

Mother found it and asked who Florence was. I was embarrassed and just said someone I knew.

The days passed quickly after that. Summer would soon be over and I couldn't wait to start school again.

*

I went back to working after school, taking whatever jobs I could get. One was as an usher at a Trans-Lux movie theater. I simply went to the entrance of the theater on the east side of 84th Street and asked if I could get a job. A very funny, strange-looking man with a narrow face said he could use an usher in the evening between six and eleven o'clock.

I wore the uniform proudly and admired the wealthy patrons from the East Side in their fine clothes.

From my station in the back row I watched the same movies over and over. A particular favorite was the British film with Wendy Hiller, *I Know Where I'm Going*

One evening I was taking tickets as usual when a group of people walked in and said, "Oh, it's that Siegfried Kra. What are you doing here?"

These people knew me from Danzig when we was rich. I simply smiled and said I was just doing this for a little while. I no longer felt proud of the uniform but embarrassed by it.

*

One evening I led Henry Fonda to his seat and the star gave me a quarter tip.

But the head usher, a miserable-looking man, criticized me for the way I wore the uniform. He had it in for me because soon after, I was fired. But I was glad to be free from this humility. Better to work in a dark room or a basement somewhere where no one could see me.

The Sanatorium

THE TRAIN RIDE from Lausanne, Switzerland, to Leysin took forty-five minutes, winding through the beautiful valleys of the Swiss Alps. It was the winter of 1952, and I was on this train heading for the famous TB sanatorium. The sanatorium was located on top of one of the magnificent Alpine mountains, and the train stopped at its base. The air here was clear and dry, and the mountain was covered by miles of sparkling white snow. Everything, including the sanatorium, was white, except for the elevator—a freight elevator that carried the dead back down the mountain to the train that would take them back to Lausanne. It looked like the freight elevator in New York that lifted cars to their parking spots.

Fifteen medical students were crowded into this vertical moving bus, which had a medicinal smell. Fifteen medical students ascended to meet TB patients for the first time. They had come to learn about the most dreadful disease of the century.

They took little notice of the beauty that surrounded them because of their fears and anxiety of what lay before them.

*

Not far from this sanatorium was a renowned health and ski spa where healthy people went to enjoy the pleasures of the grand tranquility of the mountains and the air.

A pleasant-looking nurse met us as we stepped off the elevator and escorted us to the lecture hall. It looked like the rotunda in most other medical schools, except this one was surrounded by glass that gave view to a white paradise of glistening snow and the awesome surrounding mountains. The lecturer who was going to give the preliminary talk on TB was as tall as a giraffe, wearing a long white coat.

"I'm Professor Michaud. I have TB, mostly cured, and I have been in this sanatorium since I was a medical student like you."

His opening remarks left me unnerved because, each year, one or more students contracted TB and was forced into a sanatorium for cure. Antibiotics for the treatment of tuberculosis had not yet been discovered. The only treatment consisted of the "open-air method." Rest and exposure to the sun, along with drastic surgical treatment, such as pumping air into the stomach or chest to collapse the diseased lung. Sometimes, attempts were made to cut the TB cavity free from the lung.

I was assigned two female patients; one was in her late sixties, and the other, Gabrielle, was twenty-three years old.

Outside on a large open terrace, patients in under-clothes were strewn on long folding chairs lying in the sun like skiers resting between slaloms.

A long white corridor was lined by private patients' rooms. Each door had a plaque with the name of its tenant.

My older patient was Madame Corot, whose name was written on a small gold plaque. A pleasant voice answered after I knocked. Sitting by the window was a gray-haired woman, knitting, wearing a colorful shawl around her narrow shoulders. "*Entrez.* Please come in and close the door. We don't want a draft, do we?" she said.

"I am the new medical student assigned to examine you."

"Oh, I know, it is the beginning of the month."

"You speak English very well," I told her.

"Thank you, that is a compliment coming from an American. Actually, I taught myself. I have the time to do it. Please sit down. Would you like a glass of champagne? It is nearly lunch."

"Thank you, but it is too early for me."

"Ah, yes, you Americans live by the clock. There is a time to eat, to drink, to sleep, to work, and perhaps there is a time set to die, but you are too young to understand all that." She pushed herself off the chair and walked over to the far side of the room to the shelf of a large French armoire that was stacked with champagne bottles.

As she was pouring a glass for herself my eyes roamed around the room. It was richly furnished with a dark oak table, an upholstered chair, bookshelves, a small, round, inlaid French table and a small, four-poster canopy bed covered with a red woven blanket brocaded with golden fibers. Everywhere the room was festooned with rich colors. Ottoman brocaded fabrics and silks upholstered the chairs and benches and there were spreads on the floor. On the walls hung calligraphies of embroidered silk designs displayed in vivid colors. I felt I was standing in the room of the Sultan Suleiman from the sixteenth century.

"My family are Turks, Ottomans," she said. "I was born in Istanbul."

Outside of the room was a large balcony with a blue velvet chaise longue covered by a large canvas to protect it from the rain.

"We have to sit outside on the balcony three hours a day, and when the weather permits, the doctor asks us to sleep outside several times a week, but I am getting too old for these outside acrobatics.

"Now, my young American student, take a chair here and I will answer your questions while I drink my champagne." With pad and pencil in hand I started the routine of taking a medical history.

"How old are you?"

"The last time I counted I was sixty-one. If it weren't for you students, I would have lost count long ago."

"When was the first time you became ill?"

"Thirty-five years ago, before you were born."

"You have had TB for thirty-five years?"

"Perhaps longer. I was married and lived in the Topkapi Palace in Istanbul. When my child was six years old I became ill."

"How long have you been in Leysin?"

"Twenty-five years. The doctors said I was not to leave if I wanted to stay alive." She continued to talk without my asking her questions, and after one hour, and ten pages of scribbled notes, she said, "I am getting tired. Let us continue tomorrow. It is time for lunch. They will serve it in my chambers, and then I will have a nap, and it will be time for you to take the train back to Lausanne."

The students ate lunch in a common cafeteria used for the staff and visitors. Actually, it was a full dinner that included wine, soup, pork chops, mashed potatoes, and a Napoleon and coffee. Each of the students sitting at my table was relating their first encounters with their TB patients. At first I was reluctant to eat any of the food because the TB bacilli pervaded everywhere in this beautiful setting. But as no one else seemed to share my fears, I ate a delicious meal all for one dollar and thirty cents.

After lunch I went to visit the next patient. Her room was located on the other side of the hospital, at the end of a long hall that smelled of oxalic acid disinfectant. This was the home of the very sick patients, some who were waiting to die.

One of the students informed me that the disinfectant had seeped into the hall from one of the rooms where a patient had died. It had been cleaned and made ready for the next tenant. A stretcher passed covered with a white sheet, carrying one of the dead. They were carried down to the basement where an autopsy was performed. Then they were placed in a sealed brown box and taken down the mountain in the elevator to a special compartment train and back to their homes to be buried. The coffin was not opened again because the TB was still alive in the dead patient.

Here the patients had numbers, not names, on their doors. After knocking on the door there was no response, and I meekly opened it. Inside there was a bed with a young woman lying in it covered with a white sheet. Her eyes were closed, and she had long beautiful brown hair spread out on a large pillow like a fan. As I was about to leave she spoke in a sweet French voice, "Don't go away. I was only resting. I become so tired after lunch. I was outside all day on the deck. I hate being inside when the sun is out. Are you one of the doctors?"

My ability to speak French was improving, but I still carried a very strong accent. "I am one of the students, here to examine you."

The room was stark and depressing. There was nothing in the room except a bed, a night table, a chair and a commode with an empty urinal on the floor. A clipboard hung from the wall, keeping a daily record of the patient's temperature. Earlier, I had felt intimidated by the luxurious surrounding of Madame Carat, who had been well indoctrinated by the hundreds of medical students who had visited her. But this poor young soul was afraid, shy, and vulnerable. She lay helpless in the bed like a wounded bird, and she appeared so desperately pale I was afraid she was going to die in front of me, something I could not bear to witness. Gently, ever so softly, I moved the bare chair next to her bed.

"I am an American medical student. My French is very bad so be patient with me, and don't speak too fast, because then I won't understand you and you will have to repeat everything again."

She laughed. "I can understand you. Don't be afraid of me. You can sit down. I won't make you sick, but if I become tired you will have to come back tomorrow."

She must have seen the apprehension on my face and the pity in my eyes. Finally, I sat on the chair, sniffing the air, which smelled of the disinfectant rising from the floor.

"They just scoured the floor with that disgusting fluid," Gabrielle said. "It is good to rest. I was outside all morning where the air was fresh, so fresh that it made my body tired. I must be very sick," she sadly said. "Everyday I look to be stronger; instead I feel worse. Is that what is supposed to happen?"

"It takes time to get better. You must be patient," I told her in an unconvincing voice. "How old are you?"

I started on the traditional routine of history taking.

"Twenty-three."

Her eyes were like two light amethysts, soft, transparent like the faint lines of a Degas painting.

"How long have you been ill?"

"I am not sure. It was so long ago." Her cheeks were pale except for two jolly red circles. She kept tugging at the sheet to bring it up to her narrow neck, as if to hide the rest of her.

"I became ill on Easter day with a bad cold and it didn't improve. My father took me to the doctor and they X-rayed my chest and here I am. Simple as that. So it must be six months. Time stands still on the mountains; only the light changes." As she spoke her voice was interrupted by a violent cough and then she began to wheeze.

"Are you all right?" I asked.

"I start to cough when I speak too long. I used to love to talk, sometimes too much. When I lived at home with my parents and two younger sisters, they complained that I never stopped chatting. 'You are a chatterbox; my mother told me."

"Are you a student?" I asked.

"Yes, I dance."

Her face became violaceous red, the color of begonias in bloom. "It must be early afternoon," she said, "because that is when my fever comes to visit me and stays all night until the first light of day. My body then feels like when I was dancing, warm and sweaty, and my heart pounds. I used to be so afraid when it happened, but now it makes me sleepy. I fall into a deep peaceful sleep and dream. Oh, do I dream! I dream I am dancing on top of the mountain in the cool air, and everything smells good, instead of like disinfectant."

The nurse came into the room carrying a tray with a thermometer and jelly. "Well, I am glad to see you getting on so well with Gabrielle. Turn over, my little ballerina, time for your afternoon forecast. Doctor, you can step outside and have a smoke or something."

"Will you come back?" she asked me.

"Of course, but I will have to take the five o'clock train."

From outside the door I could hear Gabrielle's gentle voice. "Can't you warm it up once? Why do you have to stick it in there? You know it will be high. Put it under my armpit. It is just as accurate."

"Gabrielle, the doctor wants a rectal temperature."

Five minutes later the nurse was finished. She gave me a sad, knowing look and showed me the clipboard with the temperature record.

"What was it?" Gabrielle asked. "No, wait, let me guess—104. Right? I can tell because I am becoming drowsy."

"Here, take two aspirins with a little water and you will cool down."

"And I will sweat and you will have to return to change all the sheets. If you didn't bother taking the temperature I wouldn't need aspirins and you wouldn't have to change me."

"And the professor will send me out to take care of the cows," the nurse said. "When you are ready to examine her, Doctor, push this bell, and I will assist you."

"Thank you, but I still have to finish the history."

"Oh good," Gabrielle said cheerfully, "then you will have to return tomorrow and I will be all fresh and cleaned."

The nurse placed a small glass filled with a purple solution on her night table.

"It is theophylline," the nurse said to me. "You take it, Gabrielle, and don't spill it out in the bathroom. You know it helps your wheezing. Doctor, see to it she drinks it—it opens her bronchial tubes."

"I hate it. What good is it. I drink it and then it only works for a few hours and I wheeze again."

"Gabrielle, would you prefer a suppository?"

"I will drink the purple poison, thank you."

She folded her milk-white slender arms in front of her and said, "Well go ahead, ask me questions."

The nurse left the room, and I placed my notebook on my lap. Before, her eyes had been cool and youthful-looking; now they were partially closed and wet. Her body was burning up from the fever. She had small narrow eyebrows that curved gently above her drooping eyelids, as if someone had sketched them in.

"Where were you born?"

"In the Valais, in Sion. Have you ever been there?"

"No."

"Then you must visit it before you return to New York."

"How do you know I am from New York?"

"Because I guessed. I know of three cities in America: New York, Chicago, Hollywood."

"Well, you are right, I am from New York. For a minute I thought you could tell from my New York accent. Did you have any childhood diseases?" I continued.

"Yes, scarletina, mumps, chicken pox, and something else that made my cough sound like a horn, not like the kind I have now."

"Whooping cough?"

"That's it."

I glanced at my watch and it was almost five. "I have to go, Gabrielle, because I will miss my train."

"Come tomorrow after breakfast. My room number is 26, so don't get lost. There are many Gabrielles staying at Leysin, and you will have to start right from the beginning, introduce yourself and all that. And they won't be as patient as I."

"I will remember the number. Have a good night's rest."

"Can you open the window a little before you leave so then I can hear your train leave? I love to hear the train; it gives me hope that someday I will be on that train. Here in Leysin we live by sounds and light and smell, because the mountains are always the same. It is the lights that make it different. These mountains are my cell keepers, but the sounds of the train are the sounds of hope."

As I closed her door I felt a sad, indescribable pain in my chest.

The train back to Lausanne was crowded with medical students, nurses, and doctors who were free for the evening. As anxious as I was to leave for the city, I yearned to stay with Gabrielle to look after her. What if she wheezed and coughed bitterly at night, and there was no one to hear? Being isolated like a punished child in a miserable dreary room was bad medical care. She only had a bell in her room to ring for help, but that was hundreds of yards away from the nurse's station.

Next to me on the train sat a student from Zurich who was also in his senior year. His specialty was going to be TB and respiratory diseases. "How do you like our Leysin?" he asked in English.

"I find it fascinating and sad."

"We give them excellent care and most of our patients recover. Dr. Jacquet's treatment has been successful for ninety percent of our inpatients. Our sanatorium has the best record in Europe. It is even better than your famous one in Saratoga. What part of the sanatorium are you visiting?"

I told him about my first encounter with Madame Corot and Gabrielle.

"Gabrielle is one of our most serious cases."

"Will she die?"

"She has not responded to Jacquet's treatment as well as we hoped, at least not yet."

I spent the remainder of the evening in the quiet of my room reading everything I could find on TB. The signs of worsening TB are a persistent fever, continual weight loss, gross spitting up of blood, and the TB lung cavity not shrinking. As I read, the image of Gabrielle's innocent red-cheeked face seemed to fill the page and I could hear her wheezing. Later I had a fretful sleep.

*

At seven o'clock the next morning I was back on the train to Leysin. I was the only medical student on board, along with the nurses and doctors and other helpers. The chief of the TB service approached me in the hall of the sanatorium.

"Do you Americans always start your day so early? The lectures will not begin until nine. Come and have some coffee with me."

"I need an earlier start because I haven't really finished my work from yesterday."

"Well, that is noble of you. Our Swiss students know they have all the time in the world. Some wait for years before they present themselves for the final doctorate examination. This is our system. I know in America there is no such laxity."

It was the end of November and the mountain air was damp. The clouds hung over the mountains like white curtains.

Ward B was deserted except for two orderlies pushing a stretcher with a body covered by a white sheet. I stopped short and wanted to pick up the sheet. Instead I rushed to Room 26 and found the door slightly ajar. With my hand I slowly pushed the door open, and with great joy and relief, I saw Gabrielle sitting up in bed reading a book of poems by Verlaine.

"*Bon jour,*" I rejoiced.

"Aren't you a little early?" she said.

"I like to get an early start."

Her face was pale, and her eyes today looked like blue transparent glass.

"How do you feel?" I asked, still standing by the door waiting to be asked inside.

"My fever came as usual, but it didn't stay so long. I feel much better, stronger, but you can't examine me until I am cleaned up and the sheets are changed. Come back at ten. But it is nice to see you so early. I expected you on the second train."

She looked remarkably better to me. "I guess Dr. Jacquet's treatment is beginning to work." she said with a smile.

"Then a little later I will return."

I closed the door behind me and bumped into the morning nurse, who said sarcastically, "You might as well have stayed over."

My face became crimson as I scurried away from Ward B to see Madame Corot. Two women carrying the same illness; the older one in stable condition, and then Gabrielle, desperately ill. That was the instructor's intent, to demonstrate the range of TB in 1952.

Madame Corot was in her chair where I had left her the day before. "Good morning Doctor," she said. "You are an early riser. That is good; it shows a strong character and devotion. I, too, have been up early. I have already taken my morning walk. A half-hour walk followed by a glass of fresh orange juice and then yogurt with fruit, emmental with bread, and three vitamin pills. Last night I slept on my balcony for two hours in the cold air, which was invigorating, youthful. Did you ever read Boccaccio, Doctor, *The Nightingale*? You should. Then you could understand how I felt last night outside."

"Does Dr. Jacquet include champagne in his treatment program?" I asked in all seriousness.

"No, but he believes if the mind is well then cure is inevitable, and if a glass or two of champagne makes patients happy, he allows it. The professor believes the TB bacilli does not like good champagne, but the brain does. Do you know his theory, why people catch TB?"

"I don't," I said. "He has not lectured to us yet. Actually, I never met him."

"Oh, you will. If you don't meet him I will introduce you. He is a remarkable man. Not only is he a great doctor, but he is a major in the Swiss army. Now, to his theory: he believes people who have had terrible disappointments and who suffer from melancholy will develop TB or other diseases.

"My illness started when I was a young woman living at the palace where I worked as a private secretary to the sultan. My husband took up with the governess of one of the royalties and ran away with her, leaving me with a six-year-old child. I became so depressed that I planned to kill myself. At the palace they tried all sorts of potions and hydrobath cures. They soaked me in ice water and then put me into a steaming bath. The doctor of the palace was convinced that I had to be isolated from the palace. They placed me in a cell-like room, on a water diet with vitamins. I began to lose weight and still was dreadfully depressed. As I was all alone with no man in the prime of my youth, the wise man concluded it was necessary for me to have an operation to remove the excitable part of my body, the circumcision, as they called it. They removed my clitoris in one quick swipe of the razor while they administered ether."

"Where was this done?" I asked in a state of disbelief.

"At the palace there was a women's clinic for deliveries and other operations."

I remember reading that this type of barbaric treatment of women still existed even in 1950 in the Sudan, Kenya, and parts of West Africa. Even in modern Egypt this operation was still performed on peasant girls.

"But this, too, did not cure my depression. And when I began to lose more weight and develop night sweats and started to cough blood, they diagnosed me as having tuberculosis and then sent me here to Leysin twenty-five years ago. You see, my young friend of twenty or so, the TB bacilli likes to live inside of unhappy people," she continued. "But you will learn about all of this while you are here. Even in so many of our famous stories, the heroine dies of TB from a lost love, like Manon. I became ill because of my misfortunes."

I wasn't convinced that an illness could be caused or cured by the state of the mind alone. It is cured by a brilliant, marvelous drug that kills the bacilli. Antibiotics for TB, when they were discovered, closed all the sanatoriums in a few years.

The nurse arrived one hour later and Madame Corot was undressed and put into a hospital gown. I examined her lungs, heart, and stomach, and when I was finished I had found no abnormalities.

"Well Doctor, you found nothing. I am glad; it means I am getting better."

I thanked her for allowing me to examine her and then proceeded to the lecture hall, where Jacquet was to give his talk. As on the first morning, he never arrived; instead his assistant described the terminal aspect of TB.

The X-ray department was located on the ground floor and was attended by a Russian doctor called Boris Babiantz. I found Madame Corot's chest X-rays, and then hand carried them to the reading room, where Professor Babiantz was sipping coffee and smoking a cigarette.

"We haven't taken a film from Madame Corot in years," he said. "She refuses to be X-rayed. This one was taken five years ago," he said.

We both looked at her films, he with his expert eye and I as a novice. "Are you sure these are her films?" he asked.

"This is what they gave me."

"According to these films she no longer has active TB," he said. "In essence, she is cured. We perform X-rays on the patients once every six months. There must be other films on file."

We looked through the old files in the basement and did locate her chest films from ten years earlier, which demonstrated the classical TB signs, a large hole, or cavity, in the lung.

"How does she feel?" the radiologist asked.

"She complains of fatigue, but I did not find anything on the examination."

"Well then, ask the doctor in charge of her case to order some sputum collections. The TB bacilli is found in the sputum and in some cases even in the urine. According to the number of TB in the sputum, the TB is classified as to its infectability as 1+ to 4+. The latter indicated a marked contagious stage, and then extra precautions are taken by the staff."

At this sanatorium there seemed to be no signs of anyone taking precautions, such as wearing masks and gloves when examining the patients. At the beginning of each stay at Leysin, the students had a skin test for TB and a fluoroscopic examination. Most of the doctors who stayed at Leysin developed a positive test for TB. A positive test meant that a mild form of TB had been contracted.

As I was leaving the X-ray department to return to see Madame Corot, I met Dr. Jacquet. His bald head looked like a shiny bowling ball set with two large dark eyes that looked like onyx stones. He was a small man, but with large powerful arms and legs. And when he shook hands, I could hear his fingers crack from his solid grip.

"I hope you will enjoy your stay here in Leysin," he said slowly in English. "My office is open to you if you have any questions or problems." With that he disappeared, like Peter Rabbit scurrying into the hall. I never saw him again for the rest of my stay in Leysin.

It was eleven o'clock in the morning when I returned to visit with Madame Corot. The sun still had not broken through the clouds and the mountains were not visible. There was the dampness in the air before it begins to snow. She was sitting on her chaise longue on the balcony, wearing sunglasses even though there was no sun.

"The lights up here are so strong," she said, "that they hurt my eyes." She was wearing a Persian lamb fur coat and a Persian hat, looking like a Russian princess riding on a sled.

"I am sorry to bother you again."

"This is no bother," she answered. "What else is there for me to do?"

"I want to ask you some more questions before I write up your report."

"I know about the report, how important it is for the students. You are very serious. Relax a little, young man. You will be all worn out before you are thirty. You must save some of your energies for the better things in life, if you know what I mean. Well, go on then, ask some more questions."

In the European medical school system there were no examinations until the end of the year, and most of the learning was left up to the student, except for the medical reports that, it was rumored, the professors never read.

I asked Madame Corot again the same questions.

"As I told you Doctor, I am only tired, and if I do just what the doctor tells me, I get by each day. It is almost lunch. Can I offer you a glass of wine? I have had enough of the balcony for now, and I must write some correspondence before lunch because the mail leaves at three."

I was glad the interview was over because it was raw outside, and I felt my bones shake from the cold air. Or was it from her dark Turkish eyes piercing me?

Dr. Duvalle was the immediate doctor in charge of Madame Corot. He was a man about fifty years old with gray hair growing out of his nose. He had an expression on his face as if he were always smelling something foul. His lips were curled up towards his nose. He barely exchanged greetings with me, and when I asked about collecting sputum from Madame Corot, he gave me an annoyed look and said, "When you write your report, include that as part of the suggestions," he said.

"But would it not be better if I had the sputum results so I can write a thorough report, including the prognosis?"

"Your 'stage' will be finished in a week or so, and it takes several months for the culture. Unless, of course, you would like to stay here for the rest of the semester and wait for the cultures to return in two months?

"Oh, by the way, it is not necessary for you to arrive here at seven in the morning unless you want to help in the kitchen to prepare breakfast."

He was an obnoxious doctor, and I would be meeting many more like him in the future. How can such an insensitive man work with patients? I wondered. But when one of the patients strolled past him, he was remarkably charming and warm. He transformed into a different person.

After lunch I was on the large terrace, which looked like a deck of a luxury ocean liner. Although there was no sun, and the sky was covered with great ominous clouds, the patients were lying on chaise longues, barely dressed, taking their outdoor cure. I was shivering from the damp air, but the patients tolerated the cold better than I.

Gabrielle was lying on one of those chairs, covered with a light sheet, still reading her book of poetry. For a few minutes I watched her from a distance. Her long brown hair came down to her shoulders, and her face had a peaceful look. She was the youngest one on the terrace today. Occasionally, she looked up, giving a pleasant greeting to a passerby.

"Hello, Gabrielle. Aren't you cold?"

"A little, but I get used to it. Dr. Jacquet said it is the best thing for me. I missed you this morning. I was all cleaned up, waiting for you to examine me."

"I know. I am sorry. I had to see another patient."

"Was she pretty?"

"Yes, but not as pretty as you. She is old enough to be your grandmother," I said.

"Pull a chair over and sit a little while with me. Then we can go in, and you can examine me. You are wearing a different tie today," she said.

I had not noticed it. I just grabbed any tie because I had rushed out to the train.

"You are as old as I am, I bet," she said.

"Just about; perhaps a year or two older."

"Do you have a girlfriend in America?"

"No."

"How about here in Lausanne?"

"No, Gabrielle. I have no girlfriends. I am too busy to find a girl-friend."

"You are a cute-looking guy. I bet there are plenty of girls who would like to go out with an American medical student."

"Well, I have not met them yet."

"Do you like to dance?"

"No, I don't know how to very well."

"I could teach you when I get better. I would like to dance for you."

"I would be honored, Gabrielle."

"It will take me a long time to get back into shape. Ballet is really hard work."

She moved her small body under the sheet as if she were standing by an exercise bar in front of a mirror.

"I dance *Petrouchka* the best, and *Swan Lake*. Have you ever seen a ballet?"

"Yes, I saw *Swan Lake* in New York, and the *Nutcracker Suite*."

"I was invited to the Metropolitan Ballet School for one year, but then I became ill," she said softly. Her eyes became moist, and I felt a sick feeling in the pit of my stomach.

"Can you take me back to my cell," she said." I am getting chilled. I think the fever is coming back."

I wheeled her back to the room under the suspicious eyes of the other patients.

"Now, if the other doctors were as thoughtful," teased the nurse from the morning, whose name was Nurse Marais, "it would make our work easier."

"Can you help me? I have to examine Gabrielle for my write-up."

"It is not necessary," Gabrielle said.

"It is a hospital rule, Gabrielle. No doctor examines a female patient without a nurse, especially young, handsome, male medical students."

The nurse gave me a knowing glance. Nurse Marais had that

mature look of an understanding woman. It was obvious she cared a great deal about the gentle Gabrielle, not only as a patient but as if she were her daughter.

I waited outside the door as Gabrielle was undressed and made ready for the examination.

"Come on in, doctor of the future," I heard Nurse Marais yell. "I just took her temperature for you, Doctor, and it is normal for the first time in weeks. You bring good luck to Gabrielle."

I looked into her mouth first and found her tonsils to be small, but not infected. I examined her tiny ears with an otoscope, and I could hear her breathing close to my ear. Nurse Marais undid her hospital gown and held it in front of her chest as I proceeded to examine her lungs. I tapped the back of her chest to find areas of dullness and areas that would sound like a drum if there were a cavity underneath my hand. I could not find any of these abnormalities until Gabrielle said, "You have to go higher. That is where my cavity lies. Here," she said, and twisted her hand in back, touching my hand.

She was right. The tapping sound changed dramatically to a sound like a drummer playing. With my hand flat on her chest, I asked her to whisper, which would give me a clue if the lungs were filled with fluid or contained a cavity. My stethoscope on her chest moved slowly each inch as I heard both lungs wheeze and rattle and gurgle like a sulfur geyser I had once heard on a volcanic mountain. I moved to the front of her chest and Nurse Marais dropped the sheet, revealing her youthful body. Gabrielle's face flushed, and she closed her eyes as I listened to her heart.

Before the invention of the stethoscope in the 1800s, doctors placed their ears directly on the patient's chest. Besides causing all sorts of embarrassing problems for the female patients and doctors, there was also the fear of catching fleas from the patient, which was what prompted the great youthful clinician Laennec of France to remedy the situation by the invention of the stethoscope. All of Europe made a mockery of Laennec's "tube" for almost fifty years. The American Supreme Court Justice Oliver Wendell Holmes even wrote a humorous poem about Laennec's stethoscope.

In Leysin the older doctors, on occasion, still placed their ear directly on the chest for better hearing of the sounds of the heart and lungs.

The front of her chest was wheezing as loud as the back, and her heart was racing. Her eyes opened, and she looked directly at me as I listened to her heart under her breast. I felt my face turn beet red and swiftly moved away as Nurse Marais re-covered her moist chest.

She started to wheeze more than ever, and Nurse Marais poured some theophylline into a glass, which Gabrielle swiftly drank.

"Do you make all your patients wheeze?" the nurse joked.

"Only if they are allergic to me," I quickly replied.

"Very clever, doctor."

Gabrielle was now lying on the pillow. Her face had turned a purple-red, but her wheezing had subsided to some degree. "I am very sick am I not?" she said with a sad, desperate voice.

"Not so sick, Gabrielle. I have seen others who are much sicker and get better and cured."

"You better learn to lie so it doesn't show on your face, because no patient will believe what you say."

"Look, Gabrielle, I am only a medical student. You are my second case of TB. I have examined you and you ask me questions like I was some kind of expert. I really don't know how sick you are."

"Don't be annoyed. I was only trying to get information."

"I am not annoyed, just frustrated."

"Well, then you need a girlfriend."

Nurse Mantis gleamed with pleasure as we carried on this way. She reminded me that the last train was leaving in minutes.

"Are you coming early again, before the rest of the students?" Gabrielle asked.

"Of course I am. I have to look at your X-ray and write up your report and that of the other patient I examined. Well, have a good evening."

"I will miss you until tomorrow."

I wanted to tell her I would miss her too, but I dared not.

Nurse Marais accompanied me down the long hall and said, "You did very well. She is very sick, the poor sweetheart, and she cares a lot for you."

"And I for her," I said.

"When is your stage over?"

"In a few days," I told her.

"Don't tell her unless she asks. She has no friends here and does not get many visitors, except once a month her parents come. She is so young and beautiful," the nurse continued, "and she is a dreamer. She resents the doctors and all the people who can come and go freely.

I am always afraid she will do something foolish."

"Like what?" I asked in panic.

"Like leaving her bed at night and walking to the edge of the terrace and throwing herself down the mountain."

"But that can't be possible. She has to be watched then all the time."

"That is not possible."

"Has it happened?"

"Yes, but they are usually older ones who take the stroll to the bottom."

*

Back in the city that night I wrote up the case of Madame Corot while I kept thinking about Gabrielle. It was a ten page report, and my conclusion was that Madame Corot no longer had active TB and could be discharged from the sanatorium at any time.

The following morning I chose a bright red tie and blue shirt and took extra time to comb my hair. I brought a bouquet of white flowers for Gabrielle. The sky was cold and gray when I arrived at the top of the mountain. This morning the hospital looked deserted. Then I realized it was Saturday and most of the students and staff would be off until Monday morning.

Gabrielle was sleeping peacefully and her face looked angelic with some beads of perspiration on her white forehead. Sleep is a blessing for the sick; it is the only refuge they have from the horror of the reality of their illness.

Dr. Duvalle, the obnoxious doctor of the floor, greeted me coldly when I arrived on Ward B.

"I finished my report on Madame Corot," I told him.

"That is very good. Leave it on my desk and I will grade it and return it to you on Monday. What is your conclusion?" he asked.

"I think she no longer has active TB."

"You are likely correct. Why don't you tell her the good news. She will be most grateful to you, and then she can leave, and Dr. Jacquet can chalk up another cure."

Madame Corot was sitting at her table in the center of the room. The table was covered with a gold brocaded Ottoman rug, and she was sipping coffee from a small cup.

"Will you have some real Turkish coffee?" she asked. "On Saturday I treat myself with this luxury. You are an enthusiastic young man. Have you come to examine me again?"

"Well, I came to tell you some great news about your illness."

"I always like to hear good news. What is it?"

"I spoke to Dr. Duvalle."

"He is not my doctor. My personal doctor is Dr. Jacquet. Anyway, go on."

"You no longer have TB, and you can leave the sanatorium."

"Are you sure?"

"Well, I think so. And Dr. Duvalle agrees. I wanted to tell you the first thing in the morning. I was so excited!"

She remained silent and quietly sipped her coffee. "Where is your report now?" she asked. "I would like to see it."

"It is in Dr. Duvalle's office."

She slowly moved up from her chair, faced the icon on her night table, and placed her hands together as if to pray. "You fool," she started quietly and then began to scream. "This is my home. I can't leave here! Where will I go? I have no home like you. I have been here for twenty-five years, and you tell me I am cured? How dare you say that! Dr. Jacquet knows I am still sick. I can't go out there. Please leave this room and never return. I can't leave here until I die!" she screamed, and began to sob with utter desperation.

Dr. Duvalle had heard the screaming and was at the door when I left.

"What happened in there?" he asked. He saw my pale face and smirked with delight.

"I told her she was cured. Why didn't you tell me I shouldn't?"

"You didn't ask."

"You knew all this time she did not have to be here?"

"Yes. We sort let her stay here and go along with her madness, but now it will have to change."

"Why?"

"Because she will have to come to our weekly conference on who can be discharged. You will be back in Lausanne completing your studies and get a wonderful recommendation for your thorough work, and she will be out on the street."

"That is insane. Why blame it on me? You assigned me to the case."

"Unless, of course, you want to withdraw your report, and you will get an incomplete."

"I am not going to hold back on the truth," I yelled at him.

"That is your choice, sir."

This was my first lesson on the mystique of the practice of medicine. Some people will never forgive you for trying to help or even save their lives. Madame Corot was using her illness to keep a roof over her head. I later learned that her stay in Leysin would be paid for as long as she remained. It was her choice to make this her life home. Actually, the doctors were being humanitarians by going along with her madness. Or had they been doing her a great disservice by not having forced her back to the mainstream of life years ago?

*

If only I could say this of my other patient. The radiologist on call for the weekend was well acquainted with Gabrielle's illness. He swiftly retrieved her X-ray films, and in the darkness of the room he uttered a sad sigh.

"If you look here, she has two large TB cavities which are not healing. That corresponds to your physical findings," the doctor said. "We collapsed the lung once, called a pneumothorax, which did nothing to help her. Medical treatment is a continual game of hits and misses; luckily most patients get better despite their treatment."

He saw the forlorn look on my face in the darkness of the X-ray room and offered me a cigarette.

"So you think she will die?"

"My life is lived in the shadows of the day and I deal in shadows. That is the question you have to address to Dr. Jacquet when he returns. Some patients live on for months, others for weeks, and then there is always the chance a cure for TB will be developed. There is a doctor by the name of Waxman, in Boston, who has been working on such a drug.

"You have a special interest in this case?" he asked me.

"I care a lot for Gabrielle. She is too young to die."

"We all do. She is as gentle as an edelweiss flower on our mountains. But her sputum is swarming with active TB bacilli," the radiologist continued. "She also has a heart murmur that has developed since she's been in the hospital."

"A heart murmur? I did not hear one. I examined her just yesterday."

"It is not easy to hear. One of our interns picked it up and the cardiologist confirmed it. That is another one of her problems we have to solve. She doesn't have rheumatic fever, which is so common today in our young people, and the heart murmur is getting louder."

This was not a good day for me. First I caused great chaos in Madame Corot's life, and now I learned I had completely missed a heart murmur.

"Go and listen to her heart again and you will hear it. That is why you go to medical school, to learn. Don't look so downcast. This won't be the first time you will miss a heart murmur. Why do you think I became a radiologist?" he laughed. He placed his arm about my shoulder and said, "You can only become a doctor if you care and if you experience failure. It makes you humble and more careful. It is not the end of the world."

*

Gabrielle was sitting up in a chair by the window, her hair now tied in a ponytail with a small red ribbon.

"Thank you for the flowers. They are beautiful."

"How are you feeling?"

"Better, but a little sad. Look outside."

The entire world outside was painted white. The mountains were no longer visible and the last few red autumn leaves were now off the trees. It was snowing heavily, like in the heart of winter.

"Snow comes early to Leysin and never leaves," she said. "Professor Jacquet makes us lie out on the snow when the sun is out with only our underclothing on."

"Gabrielle, I have to listen to your heart again."

"How nice. You know it makes me a little nervous, but only when you examine me. I love your beside manners. You are so gentle."

"I am going to call the nurse. I will be right back."

"You don't have to call the nurse. I trust you."

"I'd rather call the nurse, Gabrielle."

Nurse Marais, luckily, was working the weekend. She was sitting at her desk, busy writing in the charts.

"I am sorry to bother you, but could you help me again? I have to listen to Gabrielle's heart."

"You did already, yesterday."

"I know, but I missed a heart murmur completely. I can't write the report up until I hear it."

"It is Saturday. All the students are gone. Why don't you go back to Lausanne? Come back on Monday. I am the only nurse on for two wings."

She looked at me again. "When you get that puppy look on your face," she said, "you and that little ballerina, I can't resist. All right, come on. You have ten minutes."

"I only need five."

This time I listened to Gabrielle's heart first while she was sitting up and then lying down, and the murmur was there. It came from one of the valves of the heart, but I was not certain which one.

"Why are you listening so much? Do I have heart trouble now? If I do, it is all your fault."

"Thank you, Nurse Marais," I said.

"Will you be back today?" Gabrielle asked.

"Yes, but I have to write up your case before I forget everything."

There was a large comfortable library with easy chairs, tables, and good lighting. I described my findings in detail and wrote my conclusions, which troubled me because my only diagnosis was pulmonary TB. I still was left without an explanation for the cause of the heart murmur.

It was past 5:00 p.m. when I finally finished the long write up, and it was dark outside. The snow fell furiously with wind howling circles around the sanatorium.

When I returned to Gabrielle's room the nurse told me the trains would not be running until the morning because of the storm.

"Oh, wonderful. Then you will have to stay here all night. Thank you, storm," Gabrielle said.

"I suppose you will want to eat here with the princess," the nurse said.

With not much resolution, I said, "I will eat in the cafeteria."

"I will bring you a tray," the nurse said, "and perhaps through some sniffing around I can find a carafe of wine. You worked hard today and you deserve it. But don't go shouting this to the other students because then there will be trouble."

Half an hour later, Nurse Marais brought two trays, a small white tablecloth, and two candles with a carafe of red wine.

"There now, my *petite, bon appetit.*" She returned minutes later with a blanket and a pillow. "In case you decide to sleep on the chair next to mademoiselle."

There was a small radio in the room and Edith Piaf was singing, "*Man Homme,*" my man.

"Do you like the Little Bird too?" Gabrielle asked.

"She is my favorite singer," I replied.

I lit the two small candles on the round table and ate the usually unappetizing hospital meal, which tonight was like a feast. The candlelight's glow made Gabrielle's face appear languid and beautiful. We ate the small pieces of ripened camembert while sipping the wine for dessert. Gabrielle's face turned red. At first I thought it was the wine, but it was her night temperature rising. She tried to suppress a cough, and then her wheezing became audible in the room. She rose from the table and opened the drab-looking blinds.

"I have to open the window just a bit. It helps me breathe better."

Snowflakes settled on her brown hair as they sped through the window. She took a swallow of the purple medicine by her bedside and the wheezing began to subside. From her dresser she brought out some photographs of herself and placed them on the table, like a fortune teller.

"Perhaps it will be the worst snowstorm of the century, and you will have to stay here for days with me. Would you like that?"

"Yes, I would like that very much."

"These are my parents in front of our house, and my two sisters."

"They all look like you," I remarked. "But not as pretty."

"Do you think I am pretty?"

"Of course, very."

"Much prettier than any of your girlfriends?"

"Yes, if had any girlfriends."

"Then you really like me?"

"Yes, of course I do. I like you a lot, Gabrielle."

She gave me a sweet coy smile and loosened the little ribbon which held her hair. It came falling down her back as gently as the snowflakes were falling outside.

"This is me dancing." She produced a photograph of herself doing a pirouette, wearing her leotards. Other photographs followed, showing Gabrielle in her *Petrushka* costume. She looked at the photographs with an anguished expression.

"I will never dance again," she said in a solemn voice. "You saw my X rays, did you not?"

"Yes."

"Well, they must be pretty bad. When do you think I will die?"

"That is ridiculous! You don't know what you are saying. If you are going to talk like that I am going to leave."

She started to cry. I wanted to cry with her. I sat next to her and placed my arms around her small, soft shoulders.

"You did that to get my sympathy, Gabrielle, and it won't work. You will be cured in a few months and you won't even remember me when you get back to your stage life."

"Then I will be all right? Are you sure? I believe you for tonight. Because tonight is a magical night. I feel so alive for the first time since I came to Leysin. God sent the snow to keep you here for me. I want to dance for you."

"I want to see you dance, which will be very soon."

"Not very soon. Now. Tonight. I feel strong enough. You step outside and I will put on my leotards. Return in a few minutes. Dr. Jacquet said that some exercise is good for me."

"Gabrielle, you can't dance now. You are not strong enough. You might harm yourself."

She started to undo her robe.

"All right. All right. Call when you are ready."

When I returned she was dressed in her leotards, and she looked adorable. Her hair was now drawn into a bun, and she stood bent over slightly with her delicate arms crossed over her side. Slowly she moved her body gracefully, with her arms stretched, circling in mid-air, and then she was on her toes circling the room, then jumping in the air as I stood entranced by this strange scene. For a moment we were both transported to a recital hall. Beads of perspiration appeared on her forehead as she bounced from one end of the small room to the other. Her eyes always focused on me. Then she stopped, bowed her head and knelt down as I applauded.

"That was beautiful, Gabrielle. You are incredible."

"Did you really like me?"

"Yes, I'm speechless."

She fell back on the bed, wiping her forehead with a towel.

"Now I am tired. I want to take a little rest, but you now have to read to me with your cute French accent from my poetry book. Here," she said, "read *The Living Flame* by Baudelaire. I will close my eyes and imagine we are in a small café in Paris on the Left Bank, and we are sipping fine cognac and coffee and it is late at night."

I started to read the beautiful poem out loud. One of the lines I was fearful to recite: "They sing of Death, you sing the Resurrection. Bright stars whose brilliance no sun can dull!"

Gabrielle was sleeping soundly and I covered her perspiring body with a blanket. I sat in the hard, uncomfortable chair, scrutinizing her labored breathing. This was the first of many more times to come when I would be sitting by the bedside of a critically ill patient. Sweet Gabrielle, so young and innocent. Why should she be suffering so much? I could not imagine the world without her.

*

Several hours later she awoke, uttering a soft gentle sigh, as if she were returning from a beautiful dream. I was sitting in the chair, finishing up her case history.

"You are still here while I am sleeping. I am sorry. You must be so bored."

"Actually not, I was doing my homework."

"Writing about me? I hope it is nice things." She pulled the vase of flowers from her night table and held them close to her bosom.

"These are so beautiful. No one ever gave me flowers like this. Now I know you like me a little." She sat up and her face blushed. "I never had a man, and I am going to die, no matter what you say. Do you like me a lot?"

"Yes, you know I do."

"Do you think I am sexy? You did see me when you examined me."

"I remember well."

"Well?"

"Well what? You are a beautiful young woman."

"Do you like my body?"

"Gabby, that is not a question to ask."

"You called me Gabby. No one ever called me that."

"In America, you would be called Gabby."

"Will you do one thing for me tonight, because tonight is my night? It was given to us."

I feared what was coming next.

"Make love to me. You don't have to kiss me, just touch me. I just want to know how it feels. I dreamed you did. It was such a heavenly dream. No one would know, and I would not betray you. You don't have to kiss me, because my mouth is filled with the deadly bacteria, and I wouldn't want you to get sick. You are too sweet and dear to me."

I wanted to race to her and place my arms around her to protect her from the Angel of Death, but she saw the anguish on my face and began to cry. "I am sorry," she said.

She cried herself to sleep while I sat motionless and confused on the chair, not knowing what to do.

*

When early morning finally arrived, I silently crept out of the room as she remained in her peaceful sleep. The trains were running again. Outside it was still dark. It had stopped snowing and a sliver of moonlight reflected on the white night. The snow was as pure as the young woman I had left. I had not needed the Hippocratic Oath to persuade me how to behave at that enticing moment. Falling in love with a patient was one thing, but to take advantage of a woman who confides all her trust in her doctor is despicable.

I watched the sun rise over the Alps from the train, which moved slowly along the snow-packed tracks. When I arrived back at my small room I had decided that I was going to care for Gabrielle. This was the first time I had ever felt so deeply about someone. I would speak to the chief of the service to get permission to see her every weekend until she was well.

*

I spent Sunday in the library and then searched for a present to give her the following morning. All the stores were closed except a tobacconist, and I found a funny-looking cowboy made of marzipan.

On Monday I took the five o'clock train to Leysin. My heart was pounding with anticipation of seeing my ballet dancer. I waited for the freight elevator, which finally arrived. There was a body in the elevator on a stretcher pushed by two orderlies. The Monday morning transferring of the dead.

When I arrived at Ward B there was no one on the floor. The

hall smelled of oxalic acid disinfectant. Gabrielle's door was open and inside a woman was kneeling on the floor with a pail, scrubbing the walls. The bed was empty. I raced outside, looking for the nurse or doctor. There was an older man and a woman standing by the nurses desk. I recognized them from the pictures that Gabrielle had shown me. They were her parents signing some papers, and they were given a bag of clothing.

"Where is Gabrielle? What happened?"

"Gabrielle is in heaven," the woman said and started to cry.

"She died on Sunday," Nurse Marais softly said. "She died in her sleep."

I looked at her parents and felt I had known them all my life. Her mother had the same face as Gabrielle.

"Did you know my daughter?" the father asked.

"Yes, we were friends for a short time."

I had to look away because tears filled my eyes.

*

In the following weeks, streptomycin was introduced for the treatment of TB in Boston—the miracle drug that arrived too late to save Gabrielle.

In spite of my medical report, which I had submitted, Madame Corot was permitted to stay until the sanatorium closed, for the new treatment of TB had cured most of the patients.

I never returned to Leysin again. Many weeks later I found the picture of Gabrielle in her leotards on the inside of my medical jacket pocket. She must have slipped it in while I was sleeping at her bedside. It had a small inscription: "This is how I want you to remember me," and she quoted one other line of the poem we had read together: "You sing the Resurrection of my soul."

The Fire

*O*UR FORTUNE IMPROVED somewhat at home. Instead of having noodles and milk every night we would now occasionally have chicken or steak. My father would yell because the steak was too well done. We squeezed orange juice and fried eggs and bacon in our small kitchen. We had to quickly clear the table after meals and immediately put the garbage in the dumbwaiter to keep the cockroaches away. Still, despite our best efforts, they swarmed all over the portable table by the dumbwaiter.

Mother cried a lot, but she was grateful to be in America.

*

There was a cry for the war effort to collect rubber and newspaper and place them in front of the synagogue. I borrowed a grocery cart and went to the Italian shoemakers begging for their used rubber soles. The Italians had now joined the Germans in the war, but the local shoemakers located all along Amsterdam Avenue supported the Allies and gave me boxes of used rubber. They were very heavy to carry, but fit well in my grocery cart.

I also collected pounds of newspapers and brought them to the top floor of our apartment building. When I had enough collected to fill my cart I dumped them on the piles by the synagogue.

One day I took some of the rubber heels to the shoemakers on Columbus Avenue and offered them a box for five dollars. I gave the money to my parents for food. But soon the shoemakers realized they had bought back what they had contributed to the war effort and my first foray into the black market abruptly ended.

My father still had not found a job in the business world. When winter came he worked on the street shoveling snow for a few dollars a day.

*

Months before leaving Danzig he had sent a package to our rich cousin because he knew we wouldn't be allowed to bring anything out from Europe. The package contained three full-length movie reels with famous actors, such as Greta Garbo and Jan Kapurago.

He hoped to sell the films, but Warner Bros. and the other studios were not interested in foreign movies. The war was raging and they certainly didn't want movies in German or Polish.

So the films sat in our closet, forgotten. Then one day my father got the idea to take them to the Polish sections of Manhattan, Brooklyn and Greenpoint. He knew most of the Poles were Catholic and would be delighted to see these movies. He went to churches and asked the priests if their parishioners would be interested in watching these movies on Sunday.

The priests were agreeable and my father made brochures printed in Polish. I was recruited to distribute them at eight in the morning, as the Poles came to church. The local movie house would show the films and my father would get a percentage of the take. He cycled the three movies through the different communities and made enough money to keep our family going through the winter.

But I dreaded those cold wintry Sunday mornings, freezing in my thin coat and small gloves, distributing the brochures to the parishioners. My fingers turned blue.

One day one of the priests invited me into the church when he saw me freezing. I was afraid to enter, as Jews rarely ever saw the inside of a church. But the priest took me by the hand and I was glad to get out of the cold.

I saw Jesus Christ on a cross and so many candles, and seats like in a synagogue, but the people were kneeling.

After I warmed up I thanked the priest, who wanted to give me a cup of warm soup. I was starving but felt too embarrassed to accept, so I went back outside with my bundle of brochures.

*

My mother decided I must have a bar mitzvah, as I was nearing 13 years old. But we did not have the money to pay for the Hebrew lessons to teach me to read and sing the haftarah at the Saturday morning service.

My parents were still struggling to speak English. They knew Yiddish, German, and Polish. Everyone was on government rationing stamps for eggs, meat, milk, butter, coffee, and gasoline as part of the war effort. Mother went around begging fellow refugees from Danzig to borrow money, but most of them, like us, also had no money. She asked the butcher, the baker, the Irish superintendent of our building, and neighbors next door, all to no avail. They weren't even willing to take our food stamps for a loan.

One afternoon the doorbell rang, but I was afraid to answer it, fearing it might be the gas company man threatening to turn off the gas, or Fineberg the landlord screaming for the rent. When the bell kept ringing I finally opened the door and saw a small man with grey hair and brown teeth.He smiled and simply said, "I am the rabbi to teach you the haftarah for your bar mitzvah, so let me in and give me a glass of tea with a slice of lemon."

He came each week for three months, and every time I read the Hebrew wrong he hit me on the head with two fingers. And then he drank his tea with lemon in his special glass.

So I did have my bar mitzvah after all, and a dinner afterward in our small apartment, and I made a speech, as is the tradition. But I did not receive any fountain pens or watches.

Who paid for the lessons?

I didn't find out until 35 years later, when I found a stub in my late father's desk drawer from a loan shark for a diamond necklace. I thought the only thing of value we took from Danzig was the money my mother had sewn in my pants. But she also smuggled the necklace. I'm sure even my father didn't know, or he would have made her sell it to pay the bills.

But she sold it for my bar mitzvah and never told me.

*

Mother was no longer a socialite, as she had been in Europe, but she was still a social butterfly. She organized a club for Jews from Danzig. It didn't take long for word to get out and two rooms were rented on Westend Avenue for weekly meetings, with tea.

She was constantly looking for business for my father. She met one Jewish immigrant from Uruguay who had just started a business for plastics and alligator handbags and my father was given work separating plastic from metal zippers. There were mountains of old zippers in a small room in the Uruguayan's downtown factory and the plastic was sold as remnants.

There wasn't much money in this work, but the Uruguayan then offered him the dealership to sell alligator handbags. It was a wonderful break. We were all excited because some of the biggest stores grabbed up the bags.

But then the Uruguayan died of a heart attack and his family did not want my father to be the wholesaler. Our family sank back into poverty.

*

One night I was suddenly awakened by a sharp noise. I woke to find two very tall men wearing black rubber uniforms and large ugly-looking goggles and black rubber boots standing by my bed.

Was this a nightmare? Were the brutal Germans here to take us away to be killed? Had they followed us to America and finally tracked us to our squalid apartment? Where was Astor, my German shepherd? He would not allow these brutes to hurt me.

I turned over to the other side of the bed and pulled the bed sheets and blanket over my head.

Suddenly I felt two strong hands lift me off the bed and cover my face and body with the blanket. I screamed for Astor and my mother to help me.

I noticed the other man had a long rubber hose at his. side. The man who was carrying me took me into the kitchen, where my parents were screaming. The front door was opened and the cold wind howled into the apartment. Water flowed from the hoses and I choked on smoke and noticed flames. The last thing I remember before I passed out was seeing the water turning to ice on the kitchen floor.

My father would later say, "We survived the Holocaust but almost burned on West End Avenue in New York!"

Bill

$\mathcal{I}$ RENTED A SMALL suite in the Doctor's Building in New Haven, though the building's owner discouraged it: "Too many doctors in New Haven. Go to Darien or Bridgeport."

But in defiance to his advice, I signed a contract for the office and went searching for furniture.

I had no assets after what seemed a lifetime of schooling, just huge debts. I applied for a loan and was refused. "But I am an M.D. and a Yale graduate," I pleaded with the loan officer.

"But that ain't no good, Doc. No assets, no loan."

A man who happened to overhear the conversation offered to co-sign for the loan. I'd never met him and would never see him again, but thanks to him I was able to furnish and decorate the office. I covered the walls with all of my degrees and my medical license from the State of Connecticut, but I had no patients. Medical groups were just starting in those days. Most physicians practiced solo. There were no starting salaries as today from medical groups, but I did get six dollars an hour from the Yale Student Medical Clinic twice a week. At this time, I was married with a baby on the way. My pregnant wife and I lived in a small apartment at the poverty level, eating our meals very cheaply in the hospital cafeteria.

The building where I worked also housed an insurance company, which gave me an idea. I asked if they needed anyone to perform their insurance physicals and said I'd charge ten dollars per examination. I was hired on the spot.

One of the first insurance physicals I did was for a man by the name of Charlie. He was a tall, muscular man with a smart-looking face and the tough accent of a tough person. He was a graduate of Vanderbilt, but apparently was now the local mafioso, running the gambling scene and other vices, but not drugs.

The following morning, my office was crowded with seedy characters, some with flattened noses and broad shoulders. They looked like extras from Guys and Dolls. Charlie announced, "You pay the doc after he examines you."

They did, and soon I had a distinguished practice and no longer had to do insurance physicals for ten dollars. I could practice the specialty I had trained for.

One of my new patients, a man allegedly named Bill, came staggering in looking as pale as a bride's dress. He was bleeding internally and I decided to admit him to the hospital. He refused to go by ambulance, but he did consent to have his colleagues drive him. When I arrived to see him that evening, he was settled in the hospital's best private room.

Outside his room sat two men who looked like goons from a late-night horror movie. They would not allow me to enter. Once I identified myself, they straightened up as if I was an army general and let me pass. Inside, the room looked like a flower shop. Huge red and blue wreaths were scattered around the room, and an endless row of white gardenias lay across the floor. It gave the hospital room the appearance of an elaborate funeral parlor.

"Bill" was in bed, his face no longer pale. He had received several pints of blood and his eyes now moved about sharply, like a wild animal eyeing his enemy. As I came nearer to his bed, two of his hoodlums came close to me. "Hey, he's my doc—back off," he said in a garbled voice.

"Hey, Doc, when can I get out?" asked the same voice.

I wanted to say, "I am not the warden, just the doctor."

I explained to him that he was bleeding from a gastric ulcer and needed some time to heal. In those days, we only had antacids, not blood or surgery to cure an ulcer. "Just a few days, Bill, and you will be free to go," I told him "You have to stop smoking, drinking, and no aspirin."

"What—are you kidding? I can't live like that. And no broads, I suppose," he stated. The male chorus by the door erupted in laughter.

"I never restricted your sexual activity," I told him.

"Sexual activity? Is that what you Ivy guys call it?" he asked, and they roared again.

It was a particularly hot, humid day in August, and those patients who could leave their beds went out to the fire escapes for relief. From a distance, they looked like birds resting on tree branches. There were fans in the rooms, but they were turned off, and the patients and doctors sweated profusely. The doctors were buttoned up to their necks in white. The chief residents wore short-sleeved white shirts and striped ties. (At that time, there were hardly any women interns or residents.) The nurses moved in stiff white uniforms and caps. There were no nurse practitioners, just male orderlies and nursing assistants. Doctors were still regarded with great respect and dignity. It was an honor to be a doctor during those golden days of medical practice, before government and insurance companies ruled the practice of medicine. It was a particular honor to have attending medical privileges at this hospital, as they were granted only to those people who had trained at Yale.

*

At home that evening, I received a frantic call from the hospital asking me to rush in to see Bill. In my old Buick, I sped through lights, swinging my stethoscope out the window as a sign to any squad cars what my business was. I rushed up to the 8th floor and into the private room expecting Bill to be in shock or even dead. "You just missed him," the resident stated.

"What happened?" I asked with a panicked but authoritative tone.

"Your patient, in his nightdress, with his entourage, climbed down the fire escape out to the street and into a large limousine. He did not bother to check out."

We never saw Bill again, but his girlfriend did pay the hospital charges.

The Broken Bottle

ONE DAY MY mother announced she wanted to have a hotel as a summer escape for the Polish and German refugees from Danzig who were members of the club she had founded.

She found an inexpensive house for rent in the Catskills, on a lake with bungalows. The bungalows in the back of the main building were tiny but suited her well. Across from the main house was a large, beautiful lake with a small dock, to which were tied four wooden row boats.

She got the members to all chip in and borrowed the rest from Home Finances.

We went up on weekends to clean the bungalows and dining room. My job was to work in the basement, which had a wooden stove that sent heat to the dining room. We worked furiously to get the hotel ready for Memorial Day weekend.

The red and white tablecloths gave the dining room a European feel, but for the small American flags my mother placed as a centerpiece.

There was a tennis court in back of the estate and a large barn that would serve as a dance and music hall.

The flow of refugees, which really had never been more than a trickle, stopped altogether. They all knew they were fortunate to have escaped the destruction of their people in Europe, yet they could not help but compare their current struggles to make a living to their life of ease, culture and respect they had once known.

Doctors, professors, judges, who had come to this country with nothing, and for whom there was no professional employment here, labored at menial jobs. They were dishwashers, janitors, anything to earn a few dollars.

Mother's club for these Polish and German Jews was in a small apartment in an old building on the West Side. Everyone chipped in to pay the rent and electricity. It became a very democratic place, with judges and professors mingling with uneducated tradesmen. This is something that would not have happened in Europe, and I give my mother, who had been a socialite and beaux-arts graduate, credit for accepting everyone who wanted to join.

*

We opened the hotel Friday afternoon on Memorial Day weekend and waited to greet our first guests like European servants, standing at attention on the large front porch. My mother was wearing her best dress. My father wore a white shirt and red tie. I wore ironed pants and a collared shirt. Accompanying us were our initial staff: a waiter and a cook.

But no guests came, and it began to rain. We all went inside, fearing we would have to close before we even opened.

But at midnight the first guests arrived, and more came Sunday. The rain had not stopped. It was chilly and dreary and I lit the stove in the basement to try to keep everyone from catching cold.

The guests made the best of the bad weather, singing old European songs, playing bridge and chess. When I wasn't working I moved around the living room, speaking to my mother's distinguished friends. There was a woman judge from Warsaw, a pianist who was a Chopin expert, and a renowned philosopher, among others.

*

One day I was playing with some of the guests' children and chased them into the lake. I felt a sharp pain in my left ankle and screamed for help. I had stepped on a broken bottle.

My father used a towel as a tourniquet and drove me to the local doctor. When I looked down I got my first anatomy lesson. The whole area below my ankle was open. I could see the long nerves and arteries of my foot.

The doctor, a gentle soul, said to me, "You are lucky the nerves are not cut because you would not be able to walk again on that foot!"

He took a sterile needle and gut and sewed my skin together with no anaesthesia. I imagined I was in a cowboy movie and had been injured was told to bite a bullet to dampen the pain.

"Someday I want to be a doctor too," I said.

Aldo

My new cardiology practice included many Italians from nearby towns and farms in Connecticut, referred by a grateful life insurance salesman named Joe. He was a retired test pilot who had grown up in a strict Catholic Italian family that ran a small grocery store in New Haven. With each office visit he brought me a bottle of wine, grapes, tomatoes, figs—whatever was in season. Joe's lovely wife, Gwen, even became my medical assistant.

After six months in practice, my waiting room was typically filled with patients. Everything was going better than I had expected. Then one morning Gwen interrupted a consultation to whisper that there was someone on the line from the Attorney General's Office in Washington. She sounded petrified and my pulse began to race. I tried to think fast. Should I call a lawyer? Were they going to investigate me because of my Italian patients? Robert Kennedy, the tough new Attorney General, had made a pledge to go after the Mafia.

Any federal or local agency scared me. Just seeing someone in uniform or with a badge on his jacket made my heart skip a beat. The fear of being arrested and put away was a residue from my youth in Danzig when the brown shirts, Hitler Youth, and SS persecuted my family. Often I was attacked by Hitler Youth gangs on my way to school. Much of my family would perish in the Holocaust. My parents, my brother, and I escaped in 1938 only because my father was an important coal merchant and was able to buy us passage on the *Queen Mary*. Even after arriving in New York City, I still was attacked because I was Jewish. We still lived in fear that someone was going to take us away. Decades later, nothing could take away this feeling of vulnerability, even though I had become a respected physician.

So it was with a lump in my throat that I picked up the phone. The caller, who turned out to be respectful and polite, had been referred to me by the Yale Medical School. He needed an expert opinion on the cardiac condition of an individual in custody.

I was flabbergasted and speechless for a moment.

"Of course. I would be honored," I replied.

"What will be your fee?" the man asked.

I blurted out, "Fifty dollars." Was that too much?

"OK," the man answered.

I should have asked for more.

I was the first to arrive at my office the following Monday. The phone was already ringing.

"Hey, Doc, you're gonna examine one of my friends," a gruff voice stated. "The Feds are bringing him to see you."

"Who is this?"

"You let this guy go, understand? You will regret it if you don't, and your family will, too. Understand? You make your report he can't be incarcerated," the caller continued, accenting each syllable of "incarcerated."

I didn't know what to say, but it didn't matter. The caller had hung up.

I was filled more with anger than fright. While uniforms and badges made me feel vulnerable, for some reason I was never intimidated by common criminals and thugs.

What hubris and audacity, I thought, for him to try to interfere in the sacred doctor-patient relationship.

Twenty minutes later two tall, thin men who looked like they'd been sent from FBI central casting walked in, pulling an older man with curly hair, a grayish complexion, and a head as large as a horse's. Despite being handcuffed and short of breath, he smiled at me and seemed friendlier than the stolid agents, who flashed their badges and handed me a leather briefcase filled with medical reports.

"You expect me to read all these?" I asked.

"That's up to you. You're the doctor," the taller of the agents answered.

I was about to mention the threatening phone call, but looking at the patient, who didn't seem like someone who would harm my family, I decided to hear his story first.

One of the agents stayed in the waiting room, but the taller one insisted on coming with us to my exam room and removed the patient's handcuffs. He left us alone only when I declared the sacredness of the doctor-patient relationship.

The patient spoke in a soft, intelligent voice. He was suffering from severe coronary artery disease and angina. The famous Texas doctor Denton Cooley had written that if Aldo went to jail, he would die in a few months. Dr. Cooley's mentor, Dr. Debarked, agreed. But the federal government wanted this guy behind bars and they had come to me for a third opinion. They wouldn't tell me what crime or crimes he had committed, only that mine would be the final determination.

Aldo gave a convincing history of chest pain with effort and severe shortness of breath. This was in an era before stress tests and cardiac cauterization.

But it was quite evident that Aldo was prone to sudden death and not by electric chair but by his own lifestyle. He was only in his early thirties, like me, but his heart was that of an old man.

The more I chatted with him, the more I began to like him. After I finished my examination, I told Aldo that I agreed with Dr. Cooley that he did have severe heart disease and added, "But I disagree that you shouldn't be incarcerated."

Aldo's smile vanished, his face turned red, and he looked as if he was ready to strike me.

"Now listen for a minute," I told him. "Your diet and lifestyle are already a death sentence. If you go free you will be dead in a few weeks or months with the crowd you hang around. But I happen to know that Dr. Cooley is doing a new experimental surgical procedure. If you go to jail and have chest pain, they will put you in the hospital and I think you will qualify for it."

Aldo eyed me suspiciously, but he knew he was at death's door and ultimately agreed.

I wrote my report and made the Attorney General happy. Aldo went to prison. Three months later I received a large wreath of carnations with the note: "Doc, thanks. I was operated on and am doing fine."

I also received a fifty-dollar check from the Attorney General's Office, which I never cashed. It hangs framed on the wall behind my desk.

And the name of the experimental procedure? Coronary artery bypass surgery.

Rita

FROM THE TOP of the hill I could see the Hudson River looking gray, as a searing wind blew on my face. I was standing in front of my apartment building. On the same side of the street, a hundred feet or so away, was a residential hotel, entered by a small concrete staircase that lead into a darkened lobby, with two brown worn-out fauteuils standing on a dirty Turkish rug.

Suspicious looking characters came and went from this hotel, their faces covered with scarves, holding on to their black hats with both hands to prevent them flying off from the strong wintry wind.

This was war time and the government told us to be alert to German agents mingling with ordinary citizens. Posters in the subways and trolley cars warned that spies lurked everywhere.

I kept a sharp lookout for these murdering German spies invading our country. Surely the hotel must hide a nest of them. It was my patriotic duty to discover and report these nefarious characters to the government. After all, my father was an air raid warden for our block. He wore a blue helmet with the air raid warden insignia, which gave him the authority to order neighbors to cover their windows when the air raid sirens blasted, lest any light attract German bombers. I believed I too had to do my part for America, the country that let us escape from blazing Europe. The natives called us "greenhorns" and much worse. But of the few, lucky Jews who managed to immigrate to the United States, many became great scientists, doctors, composers, film directors, and other professionals and artists.

One day I was watching the hotel for spies when suddenly a sweet-looking young woman with beautiful brown eyes, wearing her brown hair in a bun stepped out of the mysterious concrete entrance. She must be the daughter of one of the spies, I thought.

But I had other thoughts as well. She was five feet four, just the right height for me. I took the plunge and with a big smile said, "Hi—

do you live here?"

She answered sweetly with a delightful British accent. "I live here with my parents. We just arrived from London on the S.S. *America*," she answered.

"What is your name?" I asked, thinking that coming from Britain was a good way for a German spy to pretend to be English.

"My name is Firemen and my father is a tailor."

As she talked she kept one foot on the steps of the entrance of the hotel. She wore white gloves, a blue dress and blue jacket with a white blouse. She had a tiny, friendly, pale face.

I told her my name and she proffered her little gloved hand to shake mine, but held it firmly, longer than just to shake hands.

"Would you like to take a walk down to Riverside Park and look at the river? That's the Hudson," I said with some authority, acting like an American greeting a greenhorn.

"I would like that, but I am waiting for Mommy and Father. They want to go by trolley car to see a little of New York."

Just then her father walked out of the hotel wearing a dark suit, white shirt, blue tie and a British homburg. He was a slight man with a trim mustache.

"There you are, Rita. Already made a new acquaintance?"

She introduced me as a new American friend and I shook hands with Mr. Firemen and clicked my heels slightly and bent my head.

"And you are not American I gather?" he said.

"I was born in Danzig," I said somewhat ashamed. I did not want to be identified as a greenhorn, no less from Germany. We lucky few who managed to escape from the Germans just as the slaughter of Jews was in progress. President Roosevelt knew of the tragedy but ignored it, along with the millions of Jews in America.

"Beautiful Danzig," he said. "I was once there on holiday. Danzig, where the war started. You are lucky you escaped."

I kept staring at Rita as he spoke. Her sweet face did not turn away.

*

We met the next afternoon at four in front of the hotel and walked down the steep hill to Riverside Park. The air was chilly but I warmed up quickly as I took Rita's small, soft hand.

We met each afternoon after school and wandered down to the

park. And then summer came and we became more daring, lying on the grass and kissing. Once I tried to remove her panties, but in vain.

"No, no," she repeated in her strong Cockney accent, from the east of London where the working class Jews lived.

Perspiring on the hot grass, my heart beating like a primitive drum, I did not see the policeman watching us until he gently said, "Come on you kids, just move on. Go home and do your things."

Embarrassed, we swiftly rose from the ground.

"I wish we had some place to go," I said.

"I am not doing this anymore in the park," Rita said.

But we continued to see each other. We met each morning and walked everywhere in the city. A couple times we went to the movies. One of my mother's friends, a distinguished greenhorn, was manager of an art theater house in the Village, and he invited us to see foreign movies from France and Sweden for free. We held hands and kissed as we watched *Les Miserable* with Louis Barrault.

Stefan, the manager, was a tall, distinguished man and said enviously, "You two look so much in love. Rita does not take her eyes off you."

Being so poor and so much in love was good reason to earn some money, so when the offer came to work as a bus boy in the Highmount Vellaire Hotel in the Catskills I took it, even though it meant we would be apart.

*

Three weeks later I returned to the city with a few hundred dollars in tips. School would soon begin and each morning Rita and I sat on the grass in the park while I read poetry to her from Keats, Byron and Shakespeare. In the afternoons we went to see movies for fifteen cents. We sat in the lodge section and did a lot of necking.

Rita was beginning to show signs of letting me be more sexually aggressive. One night we were sitting alone on a bench on Riverside Drive and I slipped my hand underneath her dress. But before I could go further we suddenly heard a movement in the bushes behind us. Rita turned around and realized her pocketbook was gone. We found it the next morning, empty.

"I knew what we were doing was wrong and this is my punishment," she said.

*

The world changed August 6 when the atomic bomb was dropped on Hiroshima. My world changed as well when I learned Rita was sailing back to England. I wanted to join the army and be sent to England, but the recruiting office of 96th Street told me to return in two years. She was my only real friend, the only one I felt close to and trusted.

My parents, displaced from their affluent life in Europe and now living in poverty, were too busy trying to survive to bother with my adolescent pains. Father, once a rich coal dealer living in a fifteen room house with maids and chauffeurs, now begged for menial jobs. We lived now in a two-bedroom apartment with pull-up beds, so they could double as a dining room and study. We all worked on separating zippers from old clothing, a job that paid ten cents per zipper. We also separated plastic from huge piles of remnants, a task that gave off toxic fumes. I didn't mention these jobs to Rita. My parents were proud people and still held their reputation among the Jewish community as rich industrialists. They kept their poverty a secret and I respected this in my relationship with Rita, never inviting her to our home.

The week after Rita announced her departure I accompanied her and her parents in a yellow taxi to Pier 32 and kissed her goodbye like an old friend in her third class cabin while her parents looked on sadly and said, "You will come to visit us in London."

But we both realized we would probably never see each other again, separated by thousands of miles of water and a new post-War world. I gave her my copy of Keats, inscribed, "I will love you forever."

She cried and we hugged and vowed to write each other. And for a while we did write, long letters on thin paper sent by air mail. But after a couple years the letters trickled then stopped altogether as we became more and more immersed in our new and separate lives.

*

Sixty two years later, in August 2007, I was in my busy cardiology office in Hamden, Connecticut when my secretary said I had a call from Australia. I just smirked and ignored it. I got so many calls from hucksters offering me a free trip to Florida or trying to sell me penny stocks that I didn't even ask who it was. I didn't know anyone in Australia and, being in the middle of a consultation, I told my secretary to tell whoever it was I wasn't interested.

My life since adolescence had been a long series of triumphs and disasters. Acceptance to Yale, a thriving medical practice. But on the other hand many misfortunes as well: a serious auto accident, a house fire, a life-threatening illness, a plane crash. Although I had never been alone for long since Rita, and had many romantic encounters, my love life had not been part of my success story. At least that is how I viewed it at the age of seventy-seven. My wife had left me many years ago for a German archaeologist. And my current girlfriend had lost her affection for me.

I had my suspicions she was cheating on me. It was a simple conclusion that every betrayed lover feels, just by her everyday responses. The daily kisses became less passionate, the sounds of annoyance became more frequent, and for hours at a time she did not answer her cell phone, as if she were the busy doctor.

Finally, I hired a detective to follow her. But I don't know why because when he showed me a video of her meeting her lover outside a local hotel I didn't throw her out. I didn't even confront her. I realized I was too afraid of being alone at this time in my life.

I began to wonder if any woman had ever really loved me, or if I had ever really loved them. Maybe it was just sexual on my side, or a fear of loneliness, and I was as much to blame.

I was still in the middle of examining a patient when my secretary knocked on my door.

"Doctor, I a sorry to bother you," she said. "But that caller from Australia asked if you were Siegfried Kra from New York City, and when I said yes she insisted she knew you a long time ago. She said her name was Rita."

The Plane Crash

THE MORNING WAS gray and dreary. I was making arrangements for a trip to Boston and upstate New York as part of a lecture publicity tour for my recently published book. All morning I felt uneasy, restless, and exhausted. I was peculiarly reluctant to leave. Perhaps it was the comfort of Sunday morning, surrounded by my chatty, cheerful family at the breakfast table.

I had been booked to leave from the New Haven airport at six that evening, but I had an 8:00 a.m. TV show to do. I decided to leave earlier and arrive in Boston in time to settle in before bedtime. I thought of canceling. I told my wife that I was worn out.

"I am coming down with a virus," I said. "My stomach feels upset."

"You really love to go on these tours," she said reassuringly. "You'll see, once you get on that plane and to Boston, you'll be yourself again. And in the morning, in front of the cameras, you'll be on a high— you're a born ham."

She was right, of course. I always found it exhilarating to be front and center. Even though these tours produced few book sales, I really enjoyed the notoriety. And while they only lasted a few days at a time, they offered a change from my tumultuous medical practice.

The day was unusually warm for the end of February. A slight drizzle started as I arrived at the airport. Waiting to board, I saw a little girl in a blue coat embrace her mother and then run out to the plane. I wondered why anyone would allow such a small child to travel by herself. I embraced my wife and daughter and felt a bit sad, and terribly uneasy. I suddenly wished I had driven to Boston, but then I'd have had to drive to Syracuse and Rochester and Buffalo.

An experienced traveler, I always requested the seat behind the pilot on these small Otter planes. It made me feel more secure. Snaking myself down the narrow aisle, I caught a glimpse of some of my fellow passengers. There was a tall black man. A mother and her son were in the seat opposite. The little girl in the blue coat sat next to a young man at the back of the plane. There were twelve passengers on this fully booked flight. My raincoat was on my lap, as was my brief-case, which contained a new manuscript I was working on.

Once we were airborne I spread the manuscript on my lap. From the window I could see New Haven Harbor, covered by an eerie-look-ing mist. There were two pilots. One was giving the usual in-flight instructions to the passengers, which were terribly garbled because of a defective PA system.

I wondered why pilots were always so tall and strong-looking, and charming. They gave me confidence and trust, making these small commuter planes seem somehow more substantial.

"Well folks, we should arrive in Boston in forty-five minutes," the senior pilot informed us cheerfully just as the windshield began being pelted with rain. I placed the manuscript pages back into their folder, returned it to my briefcase, and sat back, trying to relax.

I tried to plan what I was going to say on this next interview. But instead I began to wonder if I would die in a plane crash. I had been fortunate so far, having traveled hundreds of times without mishap. But what if the odds were turning against me?

My own death had not really preoccupied me until then, although as a cardiologist death was my constant companion. How many times had I stood by a bedside and witnessed the last moments of a human life? Everyone dies the same way, unlike births, which are all differ-ent. The last gasp of life is a universal phenomenon, regardless of the cause. Death is the end of a personality. Being a custodian of human lives, I was programmed to save them. This was as much a part of my brain as eating and sleeping. But who would try to save me when the time came? Who saves the doctor?

I took a comb from my jacket pocket and began to straighten my hair, arrange my tie, smooth the blazer I was wearing, as if I were grooming for a party.

My eyes were transfixed by the windshield. The wipers were mov-ing, large, thin blades that looked like long spider legs gliding back and forth, back and forth, across the glass. How could the pilots see through all the fog and mist? Then I realized that they were flying by the instruments before them.

Suddenly the wipers stopped moving in the middle of the wind-shield, like a movie that abruptly freezes a frame of the action. In seconds ice formed on the glass, and I saw the pilots' strained looks as they started pulling and pushing different levers. One of the pilots stretched out his arms. Did anyone else sense that terror was about to strike? The woman behind who was about my age? The little girl? The secretive German traveler, who held onto his briefcase as if all his valuables were inside?

First came a faint odor, almost imperceptible, but somehow familiar to me. It was not disagreeable. It began to grow until I recognized an unmistakable smell I met each day in my office, in the hospital, in the operating room: alcohol. Behind me, the passengers remained oblivious, comfortable, safe.

A little puff of smoke started to curl around the cockpit, slowly increasing, and in minutes the entire cockpit was hidden behind a thick blue miasma. The smoke made my breathing more and more labored, as if I were submerged under water. The passengers began to stir. Sleepy eyes now stared in disbelief and fear. Voices grew louder, "What the hell is going on?" Seconds later little bursts of flame appeared from the instrument panel, fire being spit by a dragon. The fire spread, licking the walls, the cockpit. I threw my raincoat at the fire. It was ablaze in seconds. The smoke increased. I began to gasp for air. I sat back and waited. We would not survive much longer without fresh air.

I wondered if this was what my family felt in their final moments in the concentration camp in Treblinka? The Germans didn't get me, but the gods would finally have their way. I wouldn't get to see my children married or write that great novel. The cabin had grown hot, dark, suffocating.

"How long can you withstand low-oxygen concentration in the blood before brain damage occurs?" my professor had asked on the final exam.

Someone shouted, "Where is the fire extinguisher?" and grabbed my tennis racket. This was a pressurized plane. We can't break a window, I thought. We mustn't. But someone did, smashing at the glass until it gave. The pilots were festooned in flames, but one of the ghastly figures stuck his head out the smashed window as the plane dove at a steep angle, shuddering and rattling. Death was upon us. I could see mountains, ice-covered mountains.

I'm in Switzerland again, in the very attic where I lived as a medical school student, I thought. There is no heat or hot water in my room, just a little electric stove, and it is a frigid winter. There is a small bed and desk, my open books upon it. Next door lives Klaus, also a student. On his desk are pictures of his father standing next to Hitler.

"Were you in the war, Klaus?" I asked.

"Yes," Klaus answered in German. "I was in the submarine service. I knew nothing of what went on. My father was Hitler's friend, a close friend."

Klaus and I often shared coffee and exchanged notes. One morning he was found dead, having jumped from the bridge in the center of town.

Suddenly the mountains were covered with a blinding bright yellow light. I squinted to see. I heard soft voices. It is so peaceful, the most peaceful moment of my entire life, absolute serenity. I am floating above the plane, an objective observer calmly watching it burn.

I must have passed out—or had I died? The plane was on the ground. I unfastened my seatbelt, moved my arms and legs. There was no pain anywhere, only heat and stifling smoke. I lurched out of my seat. There was moaning and screaming, the sounds of disaster, as I tried to run to the back of the plane. The exit door was blocked. I cleared it, then kicked it until it flew open. A tall man standing behind me dove out of the open door like a swimmer diving into a pool. Lying at his feet was the little girl with the blue coat, shrieking. Her face was covered with blood. I grabbed her by her coat and dragged her out with me. The ground was hard and icy cold. It must have snowed. I dragged the girl along the ice, away from the blazing plane.

"Stop pulling me," she screamed, "you are hurting my back!"

"Everything is okay, you're fine," I said, the doctor in me speaking. But the passenger in me was terrified.

Suddenly one of the pilots appeared, black as charcoal, weaving from side to side as if drunk. His leg was ripped and bleeding.

"Get away from the plane!" someone shouted. Passengers were crawling, staggering away. The little girl in the blue coat stood and walked. A young woman, arms outstretched before her, was feeling her way.

"I can't see!" she screamed.

I took her arm and escorted her away from the inferno. Her face was wet and red, her eyes swollen shut. We moved slowly, a grotesque march from hell. Now a terrible explosion, as if planets had collided. Then an ugly pile of acrid-smelling, burning debris was all that was left of Pilgrim Flight 458 headed for Boston. That same sense of utter peace I had experienced when the conflagration began, returned. Still I felt no pain, though I knew I'd been injured. There was no numbness. My knee was swollen to the touch, and my ankle looked black. I could feel the warmth from the burning plane. Am I still alive?

The young woman placed her arm in mine. "I'm so scared. Please! I don't see anything. Where are we?"

"You are fine," I reassured her. "We are saved. Don't worry. I'm a doctor. I will take care of you."

"Are you really a doctor? Oh, thank God! God sent you to me."

What I had assumed was frozen ground was in fact a lake, a frozen lake on a warm day. Somehow we had to cross this icy surface to safety. I strained my eyes to spot the shore and thought I saw it a long way off. If the ice were to give, the blind girl clutching my arm with all her strength would pull us down, and we would both drown. I could have left her to wander off by herself, to save my own life. I was strong enough to walk to shore. But I had never abandoned a sick person in my life, and surely wouldn't now.

"We have to walk very carefully," I told her softly. "We're on a frozen lake, but the ice seems spongy, wet. Walk carefully, step carefully."

Her grip on me grew tighter. She took small steps, brought her feet down daintily, as if she were walking on eggs.

"Just pretend that we are walking in the park on a nice fall day and that everything is safe and beautiful," I said softly. "We are lucky to have survived the plane crash. You will tell your grandchildren of that one day."

Our stroll continued, like two lovers arm in arm. Each step could mean the end of us both. I felt the patches of soft ice move slightly below my feet, but the lake remained frozen despite the warm air. The plane, we were later told, had crashed right in the center of the frozen lake. I never felt the impact. The plane slid and sailed a thousand feet across the ice before the nose gently dipped into the lake, a huge bird taking a drink. One of the wings of the plane had broken off and lay flat on the ice, smoldering. I watched it slowly begin to sink and disappear below the surface. I didn't tell my blind escort what was happening, but she heard the terrifying hiss it made and the swishing sound as the reluctant wing was drawn to its icy grave.

"What was that?" she asked in panic.

"It's the wind, nothing more. We'll be on the shore soon. We'll be safe."

Now I could clearly see the shore. On the banks of this lake of death were some young boys, standing, watching, but no one else to help.

"Walk towards the other edge!" they yelled. "It is all melted here."

We changed our course like mariners sailing the dark sea. Now I saw that others had already reached land and were urging us on. We approached shore, and the ice became soft as pudding. It reminded me of how I once crossed the streets in New York as a child. First stepping on the ice on the edge of the sidewalk and then suddenly being in water, slush.

Three young boys came to the very edge of the lake with their arms outstretched. We were entering water now. The young woman clutched me ever more tightly as, with each step, we began to sink. The icy water reached my thigh. It felt like hot moss. One more step. Safety was five feet away. I threw her with all my strength, and the three boys grabbed her by the arm, pulled her out. I struggled to get to land, the water now almost reaching my shoulder. Another step. Another. The boys had me. A mighty pull.

Soaking wet, I began to feel terribly cold. We walked, the three boys leading us through thick vines. Surely this must be a beautiful spot in the spring: yellow forsythia in full bloom, framing the lake. Then, we climbed over a barbed-wire fence.

"Just pretend that we are walking in the park on a nice fall day and that everything is safe and beautiful," I said softly. "We are lucky to have survived the plane crash. You will tell your grandchildren of that one day," I repeated.

*

"Doctor, you must sign in and be examined. You just survived a plane crash!" the nurse shouted.

I gave her a derisive smile, and said, "All I want is a hamburger. I haven't had one in years, since I've been on a damned low-cholesterol diet."

I was hungry. Famished. I felt as if I hadn't eaten in weeks. The adrenaline was overflowing. I ate three hamburgers and then called my wife.

"Don't get worried, you probably heard of the crash. If you didn't, turn on the radio. Come and get me. Bring a coat, a hat, and a bottle of scotch."

When my wife and daughter arrived I was lying on a stretcher being examined by an intern. They did not know what to expect, and both burst into tears of joy when they saw that I was in one piece. Much to the dismay of the emergency-room staff, I grabbed the scotch and drank to my heart's content. My knee was injured, but I refused to stay in the hospital. As I was leaving the emergency room, a friend who was an actor in the Yale Repertory Theater approached to thank me for pulling his daughter off the plane. The little girl in the blue coat.

*

The press swarmed, vultures lusting to hear from me about the crash, especially because I was a doctor.

So I did get my day on TV, my publicity tour, and the coverage was better than my publishers ever dreamed. Coast to coast, on every network, in the morning, at night, I was interviewed and quoted.

*

I took a long overdue vacation from my practice. My knee was badly injured, and I limped around in an Ace bandage. I consulted a physician, who prescribed painkillers, which I threw away. I had one physical therapy session. What I needed most, and did not receive from the medical profession, was a kind word of understanding. Instead, one doctor said, "You will be disabled for several months, and don't be disappointed if you can't play tennis again. Swimming is much better for you anyhow. You're getting too old to play tennis. You should know all this, being a cardiologist."

Tennis had been one of my grand pleasures in life. My tennis racquet had even saved our lives when one of the passengers, an off-duty flight engineer, used it to break the windows of the plane. Who else would have thought of breaking windows in flight?

Doctors feel uncomfortable treating other doctors, and I resented their cold approach. I consulted a neurologist to be certain I had no neurological damage to my brain. But doctors feel uncomfortable being treated by other doctors, too. I was too embarrassed to tell them that during the height of the crash I had seen that bright light that many people describe in near-death experiences. One of my colleagues checked out my cardiovascular system and declared it normal. Yet I did not feel normal. I felt separated from the world, a visitor, an observer.

Once my father had given me boxing lessons, and then I had been matched up against another boy. I had been beaten up miserably and had staggered out of the ring, dazed. That is how I felt for weeks after the crash. Yet I also felt docile, peaceful.

"How is it possible," a federal investigator asked me, "that you did not get one burn on your body when you were sitting immediately behind the flaming cockpit? The woman who sat behind you was burned to death. It took days to identify her body." These were among many unanswerable questions that unnerved me. Why had the reservoir been frozen? It had not frozen over for as long as the natives in the area could recall. And why did I have such a strong premonition of danger that day? I was not given to superstitious feelings.

Two passengers on that plane died. I was a scientist and had difficulty accepting that any master plan for my survival existed in heaven. The rabbi of my synagogue said that I been tested.

"God had too many other agendas to be concentrating on me," I told the rabbi.

But for his great and sincere concern, I contributed to the synagogue—and to the church too. Just in case.

Linda's Luck

FIVE DAYS AFTER my girlfriend, Linda, and I returned from a glorious vacation in Bordeaux, she complained of an upset stomach. Soon she suffered vomiting and diarrhea.

"Most be something you ate on the trip," I consoled her.

Just to be sure, I called one of my gastroenterologist colleagues, who concurred and assured her that in a few days all would pass as quickly as it had come.

But Linda continued to feel ill and enormously fatigued. The euphoria from our trip vanished as she complained of achiness all over her body.

It is not uncommon to have muscle and joint pains during and after a bout of gastrointestinal poisoning from tainted food. Her GI symptoms subsided, but were replaced with excruciating pain in her ankles and legs that made her scream in agony.

In the emergency room she had X-rays of her feet and ankles and blood tests for every common and exotic illness that can cause excruciating pain in a young, healthy woman. Linda was in her early thirties.

The rheumatologist had no answer and a neurologist also was baffled. Every one of the doctors agreed that the pain was related to the gastrointestinal disorder and would soon disappear. She received a prescription for pain and anti-inflammatory medications and was sent home to recuperate.

On the way home from the hospital, we stopped at our favorite restaurant, but we left before eating. Linda was not well and could barely rise from her chair. She nearly collapsed in my arms on the way to the car.

She slept little that night and as the early morning light slipped into our bedroom, an angelic smile on her face turned toward me with joy. "The pain is gone," she said.

Then she rolled over to her side of the bed and fell to the floor. "I can't move my legs!" she screamed.

She lay helpless on the floor and crawled to the bathroom while I dialed 911.

Soon the ambulance arrived and two EMTs raised her from the floor, placed her on a stretcher, and rushed her to the emergency room. She was terrified, and I tried not to let her see that I was, too.

One hour later she had a CAT scan of the brain, which was normal. All the blood tests were normal as well, except for a screening for Lyme disease. We live in suburban Connecticut. Our home stands in the woods and our flower and vegetable gardens are a veritable soup kitchen for the local deer, foxes, coyotes, and wild turkeys. Lyme disease can cause paralysis. I knew that West Nile virus was also a possibility, as was polio. A neurosurgeon was consulted, as well as a rheumatologist and another physician who performed a spinal tap, which also was normal. The more doctors who came to the emergency room to help us, the more frightened Linda became, as none of them could arrive at a diagnosis.

As the day wore on, Linda's paralysis spread. She was now unable to move her trunk or raise her body from the bed.

Her doctor performed an electric conduction muscle test, sticking needles in Linda's muscles to determine the state of her nerve conduction. When the nerves in her legs did not respond, it was concluded that the likely diagnosis was Guillain-Barré Syndrome, a serious autoimmune disorder. Linda was in great danger of becoming totally paralyzed and even dying.

*

Linda was moved to the intensive care unit and I sat helplessly at her bedside watching the paralysis ascend to her arms and neck. She told me she was seeing double and finding it difficult to swallow. Each hour the situation became more critical. We feared that she would stop breathing.

Her tidal volume, which measures breathing abilities, began to fall and she would have to be intubated. Her blood pressure rose and her heart rate increased to 160. The death rate from Guillain-Barré is 10 percent, and I feared this thirty-eight-year-old woman would become a rare statistic. In my medical career—which spanned her lifetime—I had not seen a single case of Guillain-Barré.

However, this dreadful malady has been known for centuries. William Osler, regarded the father of modern medicine, described the features of this illness in 1892. He characterized it as an ascending paralyzing illness caused by the loss of the myelin sheath that covers the nerves and the axons, called a "demyelinating inflammatory polyradiculoneuropathy". Three doctors working in the neurological center of the French Sixth Army in late August 1916 encountered two infantrymen "with motor difficulty, loss of deep tendon reflexes, numbness, and increased albumin in the spinal fluid."

Criteria for the diagnosis of Guillain-Barré remained controversial, as patients present with different symptoms of nerve damage, from eye disorders to paralysis of the entire body and death within thirty hours of onset.

Then came attempts to forestall the influenza Asian epidemic on a national scale in 1957, and the Hong Kong Flu in 1968. In the '70s President Ford issued a strong recommendation to the American public for a massive vaccination using a swine flu vaccine, issued by the CDC. The insurers refused to cover the liability for side effects because an entire population was going to be vaccinated.

Within ten weeks after the program was started, cases of Guillain-Barré were reported. Eventually thousands of cases appeared from coast to coast, and tens of millions of dollars were paid out by the government to the victims or their families.

The criteria for the proper diagnosis were somewhat defined after the vaccination debacle, but not the etiology of this terrible illness, or the acceptable treatment.

I sat by Linda's bedside as she became further paralyzed and approached death. For many years I had been the attending physician in the intensive care unit for thousands of patients, but never for someone I loved.

The infectious disease doctor suggested treating her with intravenous antibiotics for Lyme disease. The neurological team believed a compromised immune system was the cause of this disaster. Their objective was to remove the tyrant anti-globulin from the cells with intravenous gamma globulin.

As the hours ticked away, her breathing becoming weaker. We were ready at any moment to intubate her. If the central nervous system was attacked by the unknown agent, there would be no hope for her survival. Her entire respiratory and heart function would come to a sudden halt that would not respond to any outside intervention. I saw Linda move her lips in silent prayer as I clutched her hand.

*

By early morning her breathing had improved and she did not need to be intubated. She could speak and move her eyes and was able to swallow. But that was all. She had become a quadriplegic.

But each day there was some slight improvement, such as minor movements of her arms. Two weeks later her illness became stabilized and we could transfer her to the step-down intensive care unit.

The following week she was moved to the rehabilitation floor, which would become her home for the next four months. Her mother came up from Texas and was given a bed in her daughter's room.

Linda's brain was alert, but she had to be spoon-fed. Each day she asked the same question: "Will I ever be the same as before?"

"We are all praying for you," the head nurse would tell her.

An orderly transferred her from her bed to an armchair by means of a cage-like carrier called a Hoyer. This gentle orderly saw her despair and while he was swinging her in the air, would say "My *petit oiseau*, my little bird, where shall we land you today?"

"Tonight to Paris, to the Bistro Michelle."

*

So it went for weeks and weeks, Linda never complaining but hoping and praying for recovery.

This illness is often preceded by a minor viral infection. Usually, a week or so after eating poorly cooked poultry, the episodes of diarrhea and fever and muscle pain follow. After the gastrointestinal illness subsides, paralysis sets in: numbness followed by an ascending paralysis, beginning in the lower legs. It may stop or swiftly proceed to the head, often causing respiratory paralysis not unlike polio. The author Joseph Heller suffered from this illness and wrote a masterful book about his long confinement. Allan Bloom, the writer and philosopher, also suffered from it.

After four months Linda was discharged from the rehabilitation center to our home. Special ramps were built for wheelchair access, doors removed, special toilets installed, tub chairs for bathing, and a hospital bed. And an emergency button was installed but with a special flat cushion, as Linda was unable to use her hands to call for help. Aides came twice a day to wash her. A physical therapist and an occupational therapist came daily. Our housekeeper did the shopping and I cooked dinner.

*

Linda wore braces on her legs and waddled along with a cane. Each week I saw improvement, the result of her youthful strength and courage, as well as her extensive support systems. But she also suffers constant humiliation, for example, in restaurants that have no wheelchair access. Once or twice, strong young waiters had to lift her and the wheelchair to the dining room.

Her gastroenterologist, trying to determine how a healthy young woman with no immunologic tendencies or disorders could become brutally afflicted, deduced the probable cause: undercooked chicken served on our flight home from France. This causes one of the most serious forms of motor damage. Recovery is slow and many times incomplete because the basic element of the motor nerve (called the axon) becomes destroyed.

Before this catastrophe she worked as my assistant, typing medical charts, articles, and books, and she was also employed as a legal secretary. But now she cannot type, open a jar, or switch on a lamp. When buying clothes she must rub the cloth against her face to feel its texture, as she has lost all feeling in her hands. Even with her leg braces, she cannot walk more than a few hundred yards because of muscle weakness, and she cannot climb stairs.

She will not be a mother. She will not work again. We travel together only with difficulty, as it's impossible for her to walk more than a little way. Nor can we keep up the active social schedule we used to enjoy. Linda will remain disabled for as long as she lives.

Could I sue the airline whose convenient meal ruined the life of a healthy young woman? There would be no way to prove our case. And it wouldn't give Linda her life back. We have moved past frustration and bitterness to a place of familiar companionship, looking back on that idyllic vacation in France with intense nostalgia and regret.

Pulmonary Embolism

$\mathscr{I}$ HAVE SURVIVED a car-totaling accident in Switzerland, a near-shipwreck in the North Sea, and a flaming plane crash into a frozen New England lake. Not long after that last disaster, I woke in the middle of the night to find my house burning down around me; I got away with only minutes to spare. A few years later came a bitter divorce.

I had a quiet spell that lasted for many years, then came what turned out to be my most harrowing experience yet.

I was very fit, an ardent tennis player, swimmer, and hiker. And as a heart doctor, I have always practiced what I preach: I don't smoke, my weight is just right, and my lipids and blood pressure are the envy of my patients. Moreover, every day I take baby aspirin and two glasses of red Bordeaux. (Not together!) I had a balanced lifestyle, a reasonable level of stress, a busy social calendar, an enjoyable practice, and a wonderful fiancée.

The previous summer we'd taken a glorious trip to Paris and France's chateau country. Indeed, things were going almost too well. But soon after we returned, that changed. When playing my daily tennis match, I got sloppy; I couldn't chase the ball. Then, during rounds, I felt exhausted while climbing my usual five flights of stairs. I was even short of breath while gardening.

Clearly something was up. A flu? Lyme disease? Asthma? Heart trouble? After wheezing my way through a whole morning of patient visits, I went to see Dr. Roth, an internist and a colleague, and asked him to check my lungs.

The chest X-ray and ECG were normal. Through his stethoscope, though, Roth heard an accentuated second sound; he suspected either coronary artery occlusion or a pulmonary embolism.

I was whisked to the radiology department for a spiral CT scan of my lung and stunned to hear the result from the chief of radiology: "You're going to have to stay with us, my friend. You have multiple pulmonary emboli."

Although my medical side understood that these blood clots in the lung could prove fatal at any moment, I was still thinking like a well person. "I have a full afternoon scheduled," I told him. "Let's wait until tomorrow." I smiled. "I'm fine."

Fortunately, my doctors knew when to overrule a patient. They placed me on a stretcher, still wearing my business clothes and tie. My office and fiancée were notified, and I was soon en route to the intensive care unit. Along the way, I hid my face behind a copy of the New York Times, like a Mafioso dodging the camera. Despite my mounting anxiety about my condition, I was also embarrassed about being carried into the ICU, where I'd be joining some of my own patients.

So when I recognized a passing nurse, I cracked a joke: "I'm making afternoon rounds from a stretcher; it's more comfortable." That meant, "I'm still one of you." But I wasn't. I was moving deeper and deeper into the country of the ill.

The signs multiplied rapidly. Soon I got the costume—one of those depressing hospital gowns, so disconcertingly amorphous. And then accoutrements appeared: I acquired an IV line in one arm, circle pads on my chest hooking me to a monitor, wires on my finger, and nasal prongs on my nose.

I was desperate to urinate but too embarrassed to tell the aide, whom I knew. Luckily, Linda arrived. Though I could see she was shocked by the news of my condition, her presence relaxed me somewhat. I asked her to help me get to the bathroom. As I struggled to stand upright, my wires got tangled. Somebody asked a nurse to bring a urinal to me instead.

Soon I was peeing in bed, lying down, in front of an audience— quite customary in my new country, but strange to me. And still I told myself, "I'm fine." I was put on heparin, a blood thinner to help dissolve the clots. An intern showed up, took a full medical history, and gave me a physical. Then she said, apologetically, "Now I have to perform a rectal on you, Dr. Kra." I feared what that inexperienced probing finger would do. So I gave her instructions on how to perform a painless rectal examination, which mercifully she was able to follow.

Next, my resident examined me. He asked excellent, thorough questions. I gave intelligent, thorough answers. And as we quietly reviewed the situation, I tried to ignore the terror that had started to swell inside me like a blowfish. I recited all the clinical and physical signs of a pulmonary embolism. I pointed at the specific area in my chest where a distinct sound could be heard. My words were calm, objective. But I was pointing at the blowfish.

He thanked me for my erudite dissertation, listened to my heart and lungs, ordered a tranquilizer—he'd noticed my growing anxiety— and raised the rails of my bed to full height. The tranquilizer did the trick: I became confident and relaxed, and told those gathered around me that pulmonary embolism isn't so terrible. A little heparin, a little oxygen, some bed rest. In no time, I'd be back on the tennis court. And once again I said, "I'm fine."

Then my little army of support pulled out. No one was with me three hours later when I began to feel pain such as I had never experienced. It was as if someone had come into my room in the middle of the night and thrust a knife into my chest. Each breath brought agony. Through all the accidents, fires, and divorce, I had never felt such helplessness. This time, I couldn't crawl out of a burning plane after it crash-landed, or run from a fiery house, or climb out the window of Gestapo headquarters. I couldn't move.

I wheezed like the wood stove in my study. A nurse arrived and gasped as she saw me suffering and struggling to breathe. I was coughing, too, and each spasm brought with it a cruel new pain. She called the intern, who called the resident, who called the attending physician. The intermittent morphine they pumped through my IV line gave hardly any relief.

I remembered that a colleague once explained that screaming stimulates a center in the brain that dulls pain. I thought to myself, "How can a physician start screaming?" I even recalled the cowboy movies I'd loved as a child—how I'd watched, mesmerized, as the hero bit a bullet while a surgeon dug into his flesh with a penknife to remove an arrow or a bullet. His girlfriend would wipe his brow and squeeze his hand.

I had no bullet. I bit into the bedsheet. And I let out a muffled scream.

The morphine hit every few hours wasn't helping. I felt an unrelenting stabbing sensation. Throughout the early morning hours, I wheezed and coughed ferociously, as I'd seen countless of my heart and asthma patients do.

The resident ordered an albuterol inhaler, and a technician handed me the plastic ventilator tube. Despite my misery, I somehow laughed—which only made me cough more—because the ventilator reminded me of the ram's horn that's sounded in temple during Jewish high holidays.

At 4:00 a.m. a sweet Jamaican aide took my temperature, then measured my oxygen level, which had begun to drop dramatically. "How do you feel?" she asked in her delightful island accent. "I feel fine, never better," I answered, lying.

Why didn't I tell her, or anyone, the truth? My fear of death was well hidden. The fear of pain was close and real, but we doctors need the illusion of complete control. That illusion had no room for fear.

At times, my mind raced. How sweet, I thought, to be able to breathe freely, unrestrictedly—to be able to run across a tennis court, swim 100 yards, or jog down a country road. Or walk across a room, for that matter. Or speak without gasping after each word. Nothing in the world mattered to me at that moment. I didn't care what was happening in Taiwan or the Middle East.

Later that morning, Linda returned. She wiped my brow and squeezed my hand. One of my old merchant marine buddies walked into my room just as I reached the height of despair. I gasped a greeting, then coughed at him for a while. He soon left.

Seeing that no relief came with intermittent morphine shots, my good doctor ordered a morphine pump, the kind that cancer patients use. Every few minutes, I could push a magic button and feel sweet relief. It became my best friend. I named the pump "Marilyn."

A pulmonary specialist, a cardiologist, a vascular specialist, and a hematologist—all longtime friends of mine—attended me. My two daughters came the following day, and my oldest, a nurse, decided to sleep in my room at night. The pain and coughing didn't seem to ease. "How do you feel? Isn't it better?" the concerned staff asked hourly.

Gasping, I answered: "I'm fine." As my brother, sister-in-law, rabbi, lawyer, and accountant began showing up, some part of me acknowledged the danger I was in, yet I continued to exclaim breathlessly to one and all, "I'm fine."

The shower of emboli didn't let up. I had multiple blood clots in my lungs that could kill me if they didn't dissolve. I was given a choice: I could take a clot-busting drug or have a filter placed in me that would prevent the clots from moving into my lungs. Either option could bring problems, I knew. The clot buster could cause bleeding into my brain, maybe a stroke. But placing the filter would require a delicate surgical procedure.

In my morphine haze, I had to make this important decision and I had to make it fast or my heart would begin to fail. I'd be in half-sleep, smiling like a demented clown.

I whispered, "The filter."

Minutes later, two burly men and two female aides rolled me to and fro on a bed sheet. They heaved me onto a stretcher, like a mackerel onto a deck. With monitors blinking and my forest of lines still attached, they steered my gurney through the great halls of the intensive care unit, as I smiled sickly at the nurses, interns, residents, aides, and newspaper deliveryman. Those who recognized me looked either astonished or sad. But I kept grinning and calling out, "I shall return," like General MacArthur.

The radiologist had a quiet voice and kind face. He explained what he was about to do. It was all gibberish to me—"Marilyn" was still keeping me calm—but I nodded in agreement. Again, with the help of four people, we did the rolling-on-the-sheet act, and I was lifted onto the cold X-ray table. I gasped both for air and from the pain. "You'll feel just a little stick, and some pulling," the radiologist explained. A nurse materialized with a clipboard and pen, and I heard an urgent whisper: "We forgot to have him sign the release!"

With a system full of morphine, I would blithely have released all my assets to my ex-wife—or her lawyer, for that matter. So much for informed consent! I signed happily, and the radiologist expertly threaded the filter up my leg and into the vein of my heart, the inferior vena cava.

The following day, the crushing chest pain began to subside. They wheeled Marilyn out of the room. Seven days later, I left the hospital. Two weeks after that, I went back to my office, and three weeks later, I resumed playing tennis and swimming.

My consultants were still scratching their heads about the source of so many clots. The consensus was that they must have resulted from my plane ride home from Paris, as long periods of time sitting still are frequent triggers for clots. I'd taken all the precautions: aspirin before the trip, hourly walks during the flight, no alcohol, a lot of fluids. I even wore elastic stockings, as I'd done on much longer flights to Australia and Antarctica.

The network of professionals around me applauded my internist's astute examination, which probably saved my life. If I'd been a king, I wouldn't have received better, kinder care and attention from the house staff, doctors, nurses, aides, and secretaries.

Our medical system gets a lot of criticism, and of course it has problems. But as an expert on real trouble, I can attest to this: during my moment of greatest crisis, the system worked for me, start to finish. As a doctor, I'm proud. As a patient, I'm grateful—and a little humbled to have learned how easy it is, when you're frightened and hurting, to hide behind a wall of denial.

As thankful as I am for the care I received, in some ways I've been on high alert ever since. My own travails and those of the people around me have continued in waves of crisis and relief.

❖ Epilogue ❖

$\mathcal{I}$ STARTED THIS true tale in my father's office, sitting at his desk after he died, reminiscing. And now I've finally finished it at the age of ninety. A tale, or tales, of surviving; fighting off the devil who was waiting in the wings of Hell to grab me.

Now look at me, I still have a full head of hair and a magnificent looking face that young women still enjoy looking at! I'm like Dorian Gray minus the Evil Soul. I am not like Faust making a deal with the Devil. I can still play tennis and teach Medicine at Yale and Quinnipiac medical schools. My hearing is good, filled with the sounds of laughter and love, and even hate, for yes I hate people who are insincere and who perpetrate injustice, people who are extremely wealthy and not touched by the trammels of the world, who dance around the raindrops and never get wet. There is a shield around them that they take for granted. George Bernard Shaw said that poverty is a crime against humanity.

Many wealthy have suffered persecution, like my parents and all their generation of Jews of Europe. Many have risen from rags to riches on the cold but optimistic streets of New York. But few have fallen into poverty and pulled their way back up again. That is my story and, along with my medical acumen, it has given me a unique perspective on life.

As I write my final chapter, like so many of us who have reached this time in their lives, I have regrets, and like many I regret the things I never got to do: to learn to play golf, to learn a musical instrument, to ride a horse. But otherwise I have much to be grateful for. I have been loved, and really loved, not once but many times by beautiful women, and that's no regret. I have survived, not once but many times, the fate of those less fortunate, and that is no regret either.

So I leave this to you, Dear Reader: find love you can depend on, and as the song says: "Once you find her never let her go."

ALSO BY DR. SIEGFRIED KRA

Dancer in the Garden
2nd Edition; *The Collected Stories from a Doctor's Notebook,* Pleasure Boat Studio, 2020

❖

Twilight in Danzig
Second Edition, A Novel / Historical Fiction, Pleasure Boat Studio, 2018

❖

Twilight in Danzig: A Privileged Jewish Childhood During the Third Reich
First Edition, Nonfiction / Autobiography, Canal House, 2015

❖

The Collected Stories from a Doctor's Notebook
1st Edition; CreateSpace Independent Publishing, 2014

❖

**How to Keep Your Husband Alive: An Empowerment Tool
for Women Who Care About Their Man's Health**
Lebhar-Friedman, 2001

❖

Physical Diagnosis: A Concise Textbook
Elsevier Science Ltd, 1987

❖

**What Every Woman Must Know About Heart Disease:
A No-nonsense Approach to Diagnosing, Treating,
and Preventing the #1 Killer of Women**
Grand Central Publishing, 1997

❖

Coronary Bypass Surgery: Who Needs It
W W Norton & Co Inc, 1987

❖

Aging Myths: Reversible Causes of Mind and Memory Loss
McGraw-Hill, 1986

❖

The Good Heart Diet Cook Book
Ellen Stern, Jonathan Michaels & Siegfried J. Kra, Ticknor and Fields, 1982

❖

Examine Your Doctor: A patient's guide to avoiding medical mishaps
Houghton Mifflin Co International Inc., 1984

❖

Is Surgery Necessary?
Macmillan, 1981

❖

The Three-Legged Stallion: And Other Tales
W. W. Norton and Company, Inc., 1980

❖

**Basic Correlative Echocardiography
Technique and Interpretation**
Medical Examination Publishing Company; 2nd edition, 1977

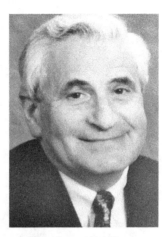

Siegfried Kra

was born in Danzig in 1930. After escaping from the Gestapo, his family emigrated to New York, where Siegfried learned how to speak English without an accent, to be viewed as an American, rather than a German. He attended CCNY, then went to medical school in France and Switzerland before completing his training in cardiology at Yale. In a half century of practice, he treated tens of thousands of patients, some of whom inspired his fictional story collections. Dr. Kra has published over a dozen books, including *What Every Woman Must Know About Heart Disease* from Warner Books, and *The Three-Legged Stallion* from W.W. Norton; and most recently from Pleasure Boat Studio, *Twilight in Danzig* and *The Dancer in the Garden*. His passions include opera, growing orchids, and tennis, which he still plays weekly at age ninety. He also still teaches as an Associate Professor of Medicine at Yale University School of Medicine and at Quinnipiac University Netter School of Medicine.

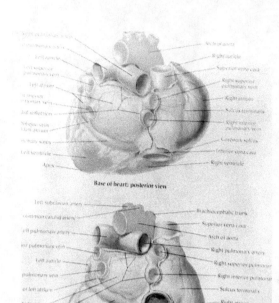

Base of heart: posterior view

A medical textbook diagram representing the chalk drawings on Kra's ceiling. Unfortunately, no pictures were taken when he was young, as he didn't own a camera.

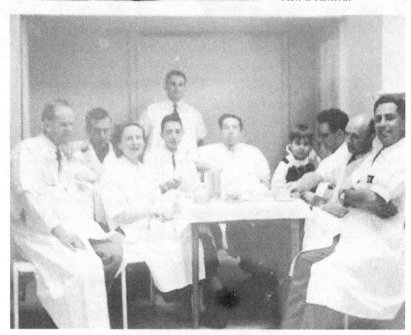

Medical Students, Dr. Kra is standing in the back.

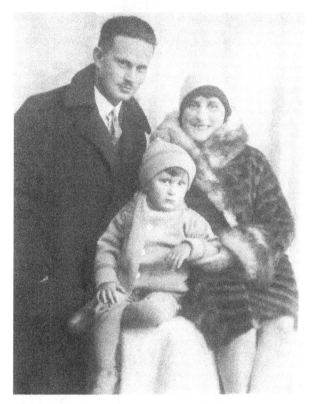

Siegfried with his parents, Mr. Henry & Mrs. Lucy Kra.

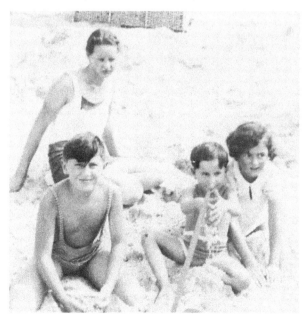

Dr. Kra with his governess.

CPSIA information can be obtained
at www.ICGtesting.com
Printed in the USA
JSHW031424201220
10436JS00001B/42

9 780912 887661